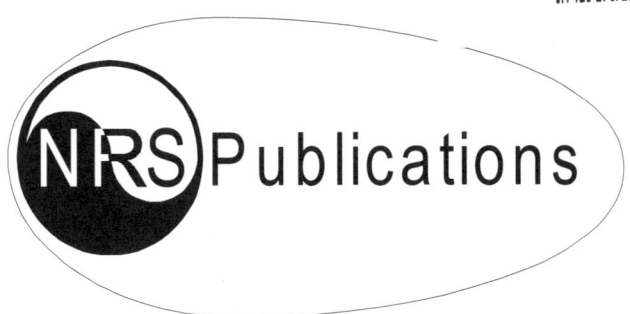

Brain Foods, Brain Poisons
is a product of the
NRS Publications Education Series

Please see our website for
updates on new publications
and seminars
www.nutritionreviewservice.com.au

I dedicate this book to all the children of the past, present and future.
Thank you for teaching us grownup's what love really is.

Title: Brain Foods, Brain Poisons : Autism as a Case in Point
ISBN 0-9756920-6-2

Brain Foods, Brain Poisons

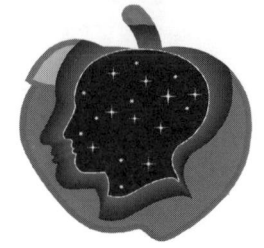

Many research groups around the planet have challenged the misconception by mainstream medicine that Autism is just a mental illness. Even with hard evidence from Immunology and Gastroenterology, the idea that Autism is a systemic disease has been totally ignored by Paediatricians and Psychiatrists. The most contentious issues arise from the evidence that toxic insults with heavy metals either cause this disease or add to the vulnerability to it.

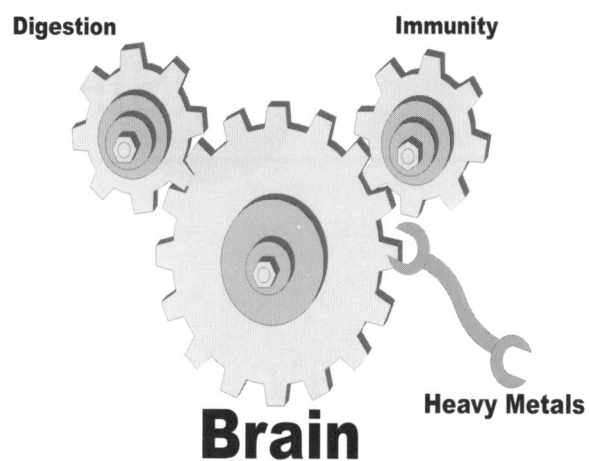

It is possible to sub classify the Metabolic observations into several parts which I will deal with one by one.

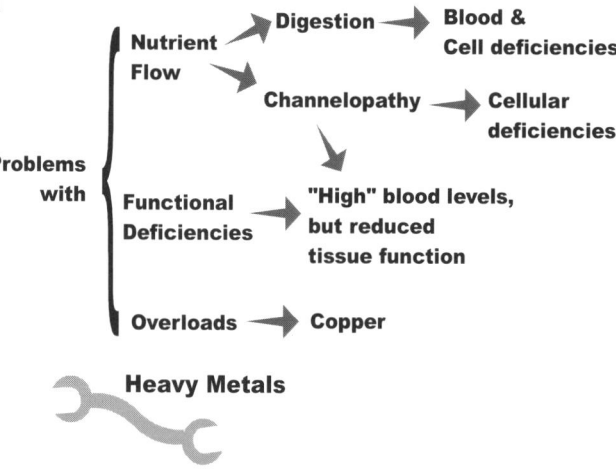

Purely on a numbers basis, we see that key nutrients have drifted out of the optimal ranges. What's surprising is the finding of both low and high levels.

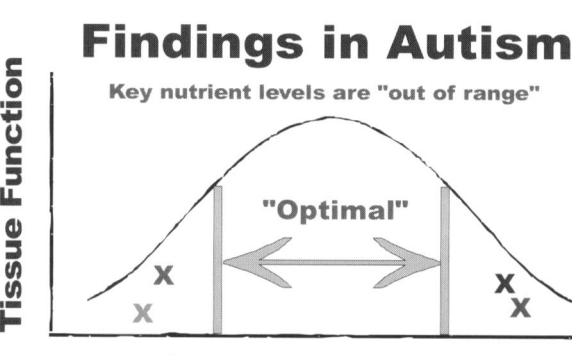

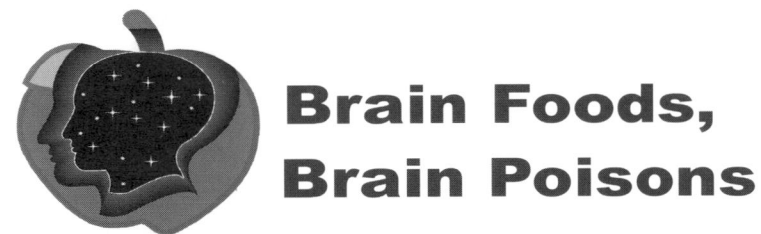

Brain Foods, Brain Poisons

Generates symptoms

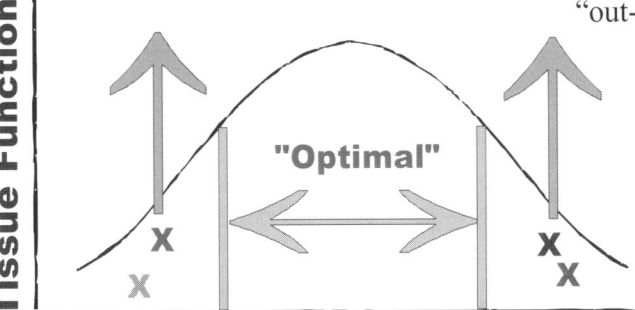

Tissue Function *(vertical axis)*

"Optimal"

X
X
X
X

Nutrient Levels

Orthomolecular Medicine believes that it is the "out-of-range" nutrients that generates symptoms.

The 'Bottom line"

Nutrient not there

Nutrient Flow
{ Low in Environment
Low in food
Poor absorption
Pre-cellular wastage
Channelopathy

Nutrient ineffective

Nutrient Blockade
{ Toxic elements
Drugs

DOM (Diagnostic Orthomolecular Medicine) simplifies the generation of symptoms into two categories. Either the nutrient *isn't there*, or it is *ineffective*. Within these categories there are further subgroups.

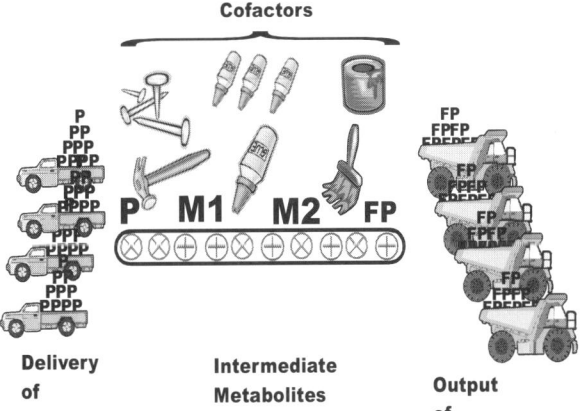

Cofactors

P   M1   M2   FP

Delivery
of
Precursor

Intermediate
Metabolites

Output
of
Final Product

Tryptophan

Serotonin

The importance of the distinction is apparent when thinking of biochemical pathways. If we take Serotonin for example, the delivery of precursors (raw materials) to the "conveyor belt" is just as important as the availability and correct function of the cofactors (recyclable tools) needed by the belt.

Brain Foods, Brain Poisons

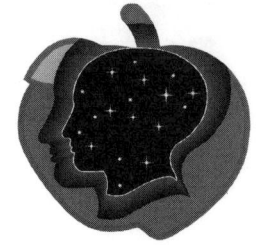

In the case of Zinc, this mineral plays several roles in brain function, sometimes as a cofactor and sometimes as a means to deliver precursors from our food to another tissue.

Zinc and Brain function

Alertness (Hypoglycaemia and Noradrenaline)

Abstract thinking

Multi-tasking

Mood

Memory

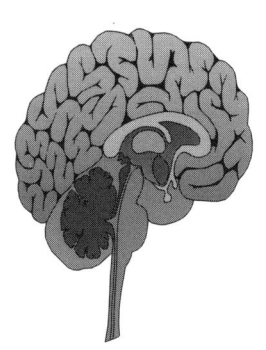

Observations of Wheat/Dairy

A ubiquitous observation is that reducing dairy and wheat intake also reduces (but not necessarily eliminates) Autistic symptoms.

Severity of Autistic symptoms

Wheat and Dairy Intake

Autism Spectrum Disorder

So then if we collate the 3 sets of observations, we can see that the majority of current research could be pigeon holed into one of the 3 groups.

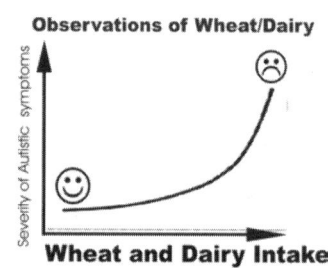

Findings in Autism Patients

Tissue Function

"Optimal"

X
X   X
                     X

Nutrient Levels

Observations of Wheat/Dairy

Severity of Autistic symptoms

Wheat and Dairy Intake

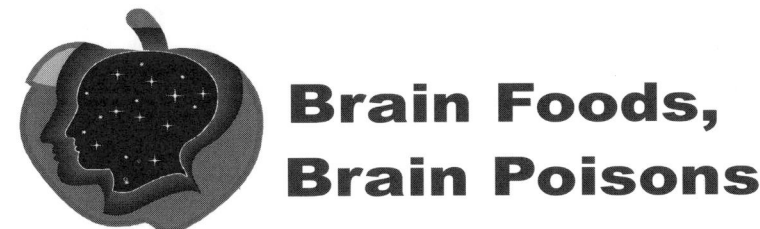

Brain Foods, Brain Poisons

DAN! reactionist approach

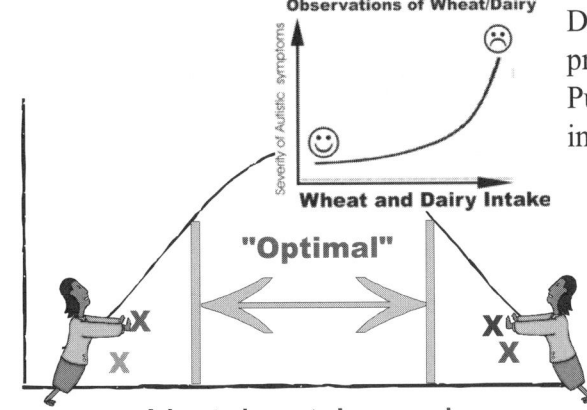

DAN! and other "think tanks" have provided protocols for "correcting" the abnormalities. Push nutrients back into range and reduce toxic insults from the environment.

Metabolic observations in Autism

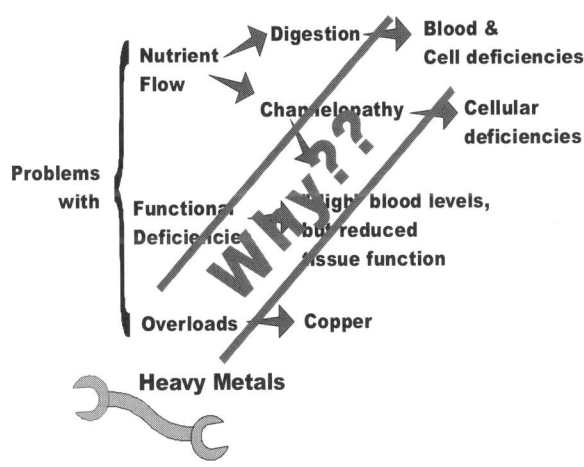

DOM would ask "why" are these abnormalities occurring? You might say this is a petty point, but I pose this question. It has been observed that severe Autistics have trouble excreting the Mercury they have. Despite Mercury removal they may not improve. Could it be that the symptoms are due to the *reason* they can't excrete Mercury, rather than the Mercury itself?

And so DOM looks for the **process** that drives nutrients out of range and attempts to explain illness by this process rather than just than ascribing illness purely to observed metabolic changes.

DOM investigative approach

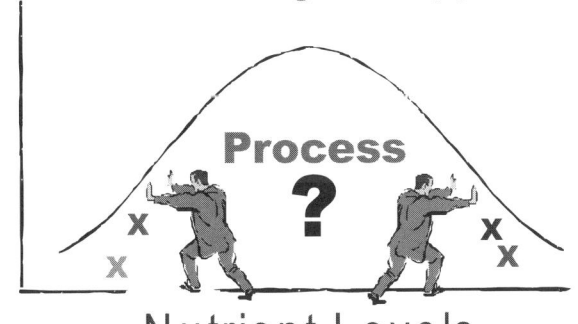

Brain Foods, Brain Poisons

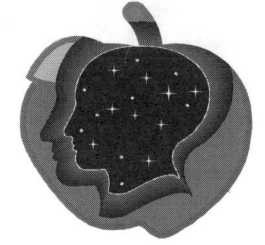

If we take the first set of observations, low levels of cell or blood nutrients come under the DOM heading of nutrient flow. In some case of Autism, the process of digestion is serverely impaired.

Metabolic observations in Autism

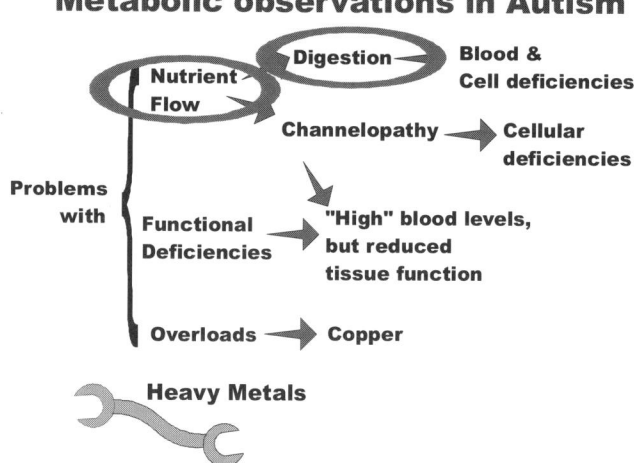

The mineral that has most impact on digestion seems to be Zinc.

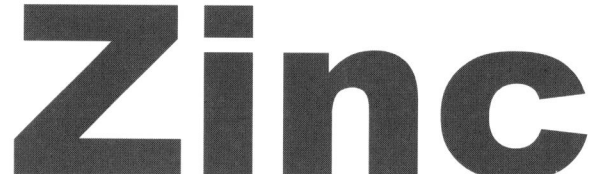

Because zinc is required for many digestive processes, low levels will affect other minerals.

Zinc is needed to make stomach acid to help absorb Iron, Calcium, Magnesium & Amino acids

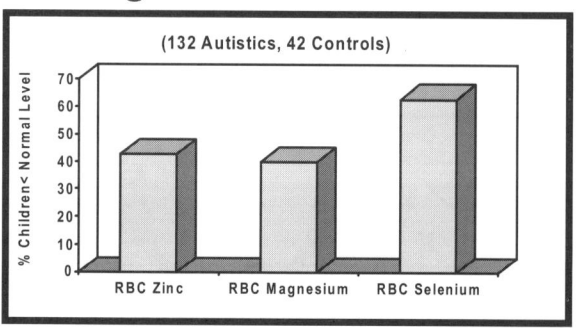

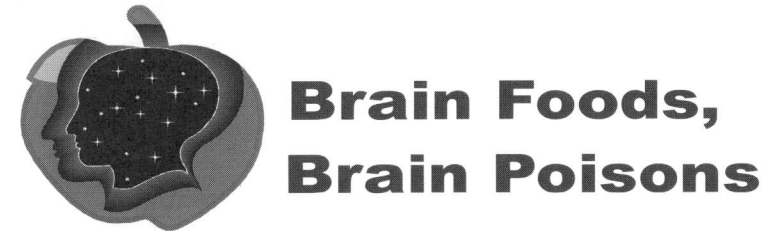

Brain Foods, Brain Poisons

Findings in Zinc deficiency

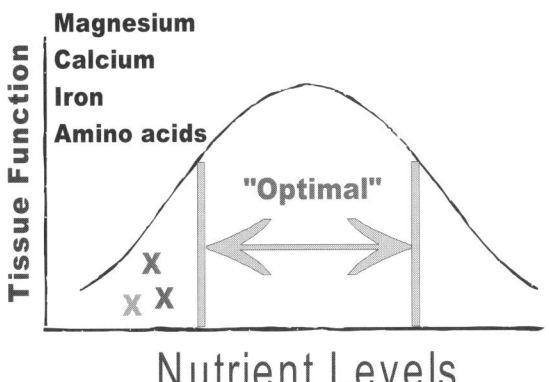

Therefore it is no surprise (in DOM terms) to find low levels of Magnesium, Calcium Iron and Amino Acids in Zinc deficiency. We see then that just Zinc deficiency explains half of the "out-of-range" nutrients. That is, Zinc deficiency explains half of the picture.

Lack of Zinc may be due to Zinc deficiency or Zinc blockade

But DOM would ask is the Zinc deficient or just not working properly?

Metal Antagonism

Mercury to Zinc **1000:1**

Cadmium to Zinc **100:1**

Copper to Zinc **6:1**

The antagonism by other metals can be measured and boiled down to simple equations. Mercury is 1000:1, Cadmium 100:1 and Copper overload 6:1. That means that the Zinc level is meaningless without knowing the levels of the other 3 metals.

Brain Foods, Brain Poisons

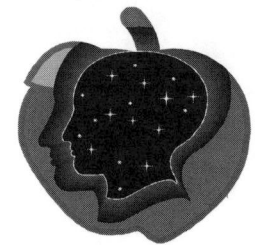

In terms of nutrient flow, all nutrients have to cross several hurdles in order to get from the environment into the cells.

Nutrient flow

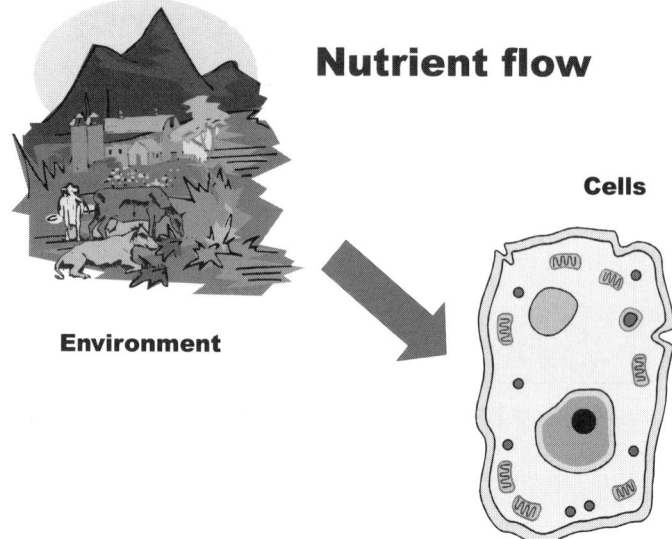

Environment

Cells

The sources of Zinc for a baby are Milk and Solids.

Sources of Zinc for a child are Milk and Food

Zinc in breast milk

Surprising to most who have seen this graph is that Zinc is the most prevalent mineral in breast milk! Zinc is important for growth (just as in plants!) and so it is the perfect mineral to stimulate this process in an infant.

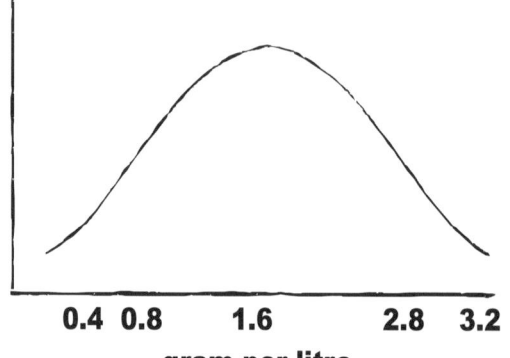

0.4 0.8   1.6   2.8 3.2
gram per litre

Range 0.2 to 3.4 + microgram/ml

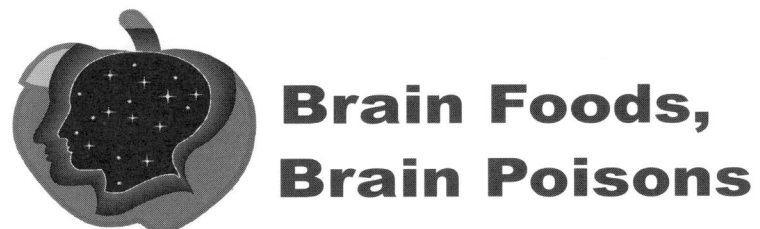

Brain Foods, Brain Poisons

Zinc as a defence shield

But Zinc also has other functions that can be likened to a defence shield. It protects us from physical stress, mental stress, infections and toxins.

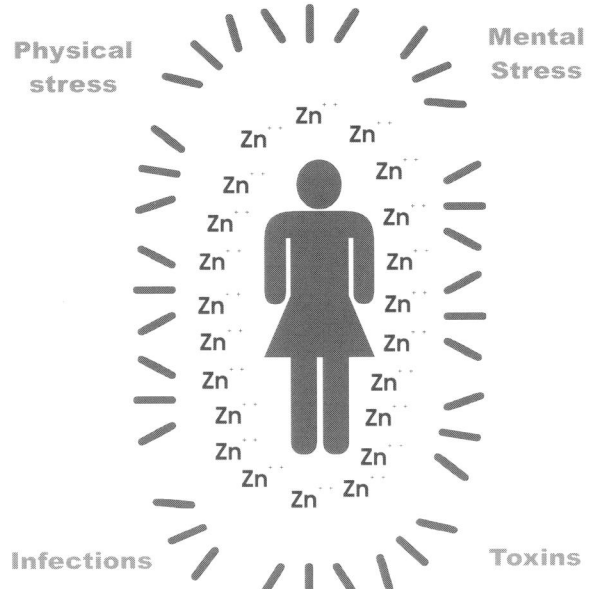

Physical stress

Mental Stress

Infections

Toxins

It forms part of the "Antioxidant Defence Shield" that protects us and our unborn children. It has been shown that the levels of antioxidants in the mother's diet prenatally affect the chance of her child getting Leukaemia.

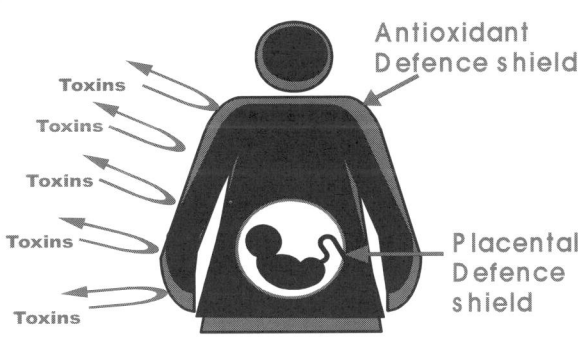

Toxins
Toxins
Toxins
Toxins
Toxins

Antioxidant Defence shield

Placental Defence shield

Zinc and secretions

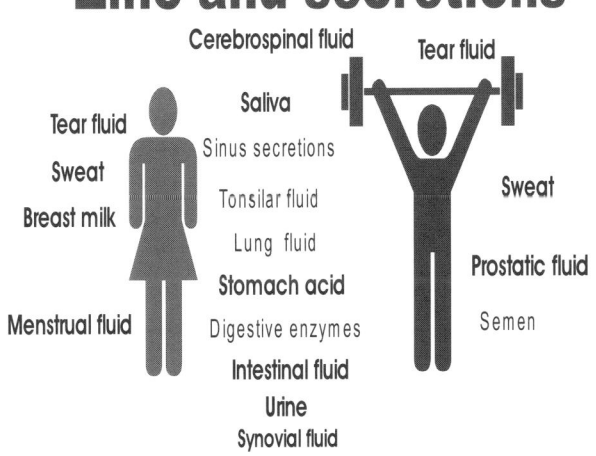

Cerebrospinal fluid
Tear fluid
Saliva
Tear fluid
Sinus secretions
Sweat
Tonsilar fluid
Breast milk
Lung fluid
Sweat
Stomach acid
Prostatic fluid
Menstrual fluid
Digestive enzymes
Semen
Intestinal fluid
Urine
Synovial fluid

One of its defence functions is in topical immunity; the significance mostly lost on the Medical profession. Zinc has anti-viral, anti-bacterial and anti-fungal properties; it is also a lubricant. When we secrete something we are opening a portal to the outside, which creates an opportunity for organisms to invade us. So the prefect mineral to put in such portals is zinc. This zinc is lost if it secreted from the skin or genital areas, but it is recycled in the digestive tract (hopefully).

9

Brain Foods, Brain Poisons

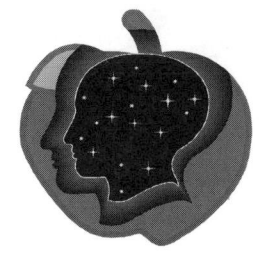

The cycle of digestion includes the role of Zinc in Hydrochloric Acid production, which is needed to ionise metals like Calcium, Iron and Magnesium into "two-plus" charge in order to absorb them in the intestine. When the stomach makes acid it sends a message to the pancreas to release pancreatic enzymes, which help digest proteins so we can absorb Amino Acids. The stomach acid permanently denatures larger proteins so that pancreatic enzymes can act more efficiently. The process of digestion is to disable immunogenic proteins and peptides (fragments of proteins) into inert, safe-to-absorb Amino Acids. The pancreas releases picolinate (made by the liver and kidney from tryptophan) into the bile to "get back the Zinc" and absorb new dietary Zinc.

In the case of the stomach, Zinc is required for acid production, but when you think about it, how come you can eat Tripe, but you don't digest your own stomach? The answer is that we have mucus layer to protect us from the acid; it is a gel layer of Zinc bicarbonate (which also needs Zinc to produce!) Zinc is required for several intestinal gland enzymes like Aminopeptidase and Carboxypeptidase and is secreted into the intestinal lumen.

Zinc, stomach acid & protein digestion

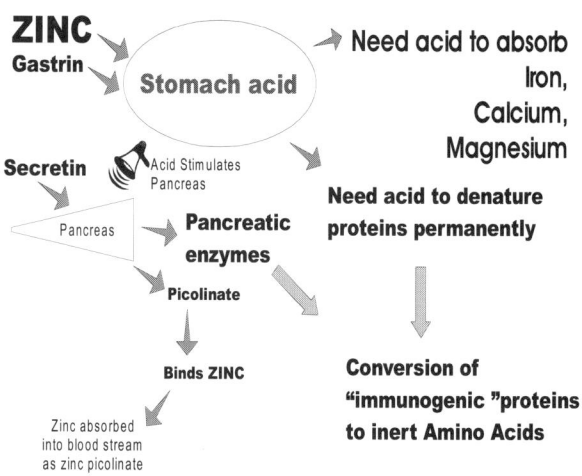

Normal Gastric lining

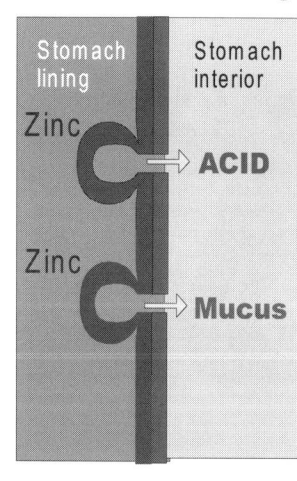

Zinc secretion into intestine

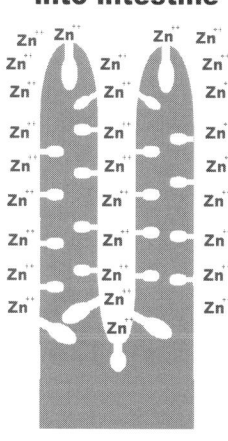

The protective role of Stomach acid has also been forgotten by medicine (which is so intent on purveying drugs that suppress stomach acid). The acid is there to destroy would be invaders, and to render harmless salicylates (natural and pharmaceutical) Food colourings, preservatives as well as proteins.

Protective Role of Stomach Acid via Zinc

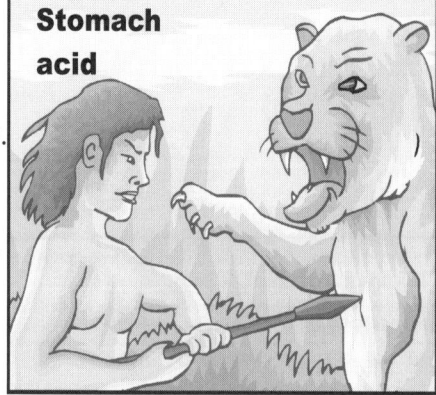

Bacteria
Viruses
Yeasts
Preservatives
Food Colourings
Salicylates
Foreign Proteins

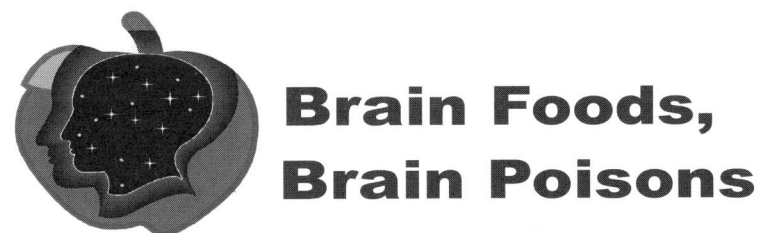

Brain Foods, Brain Poisons

Atrophic Gastric lining

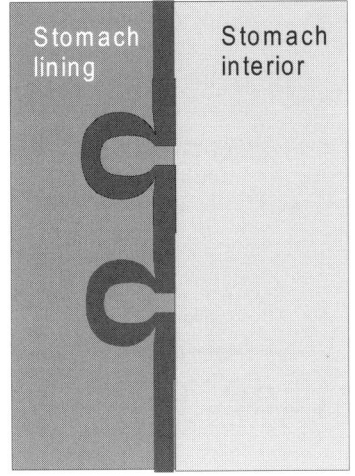

Stomach lining

Stomach interior

No acid & No mucus

So let's imagine a stomach without Zinc. No Zinc, no acid. No Zinc no mucus layer. We have the ironic situation that we need acid to digest our food, but if we have something acidic, we don't feel so well. Giving drugs to suppress stomach acid only hides the problem, and makes someone lots of money.

Zinc the wonder mineral

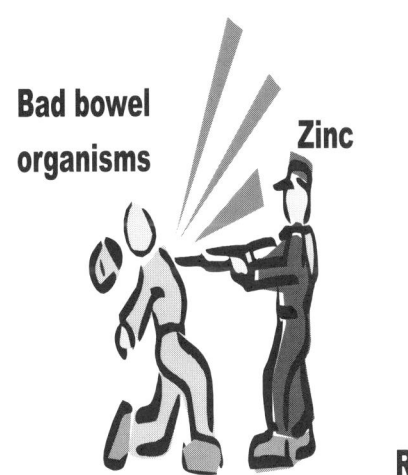

Bad bowel organisms

Zinc

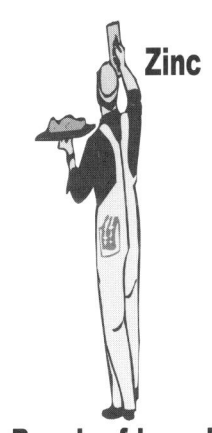

Zinc

Repair of bowel wall

The antimicrobial properties of Zinc make it ideal as a bowel bug policeman, and keeps the chance of dysbiosis very low. Zinc is needed for the repair of damaged tissue (low Zinc, delayed would healing, recurrent infections etc). So this wonder mineral makes sure that the whole intestinal tract is in good repair.

Endoscopic observations in zinc deficiency

What would happen to the gut if zinc were low? We'd get inflammation and ulcers at any point along it (including the mouth). Guess what abnormalities we see when endoscope Autism patients? Just a mental illness?

1] Oesophagitis/ulcers
2] Gastritis/ ulcers
3] Duodenitis/ulcers
4] Enteritis/ulcers
5] Colitis/ulcers

Brain Foods, Brain Poisons

Findings in Zinc deficiency

So in summary we can see that low Zinc will lead to low levels of key nutrients.

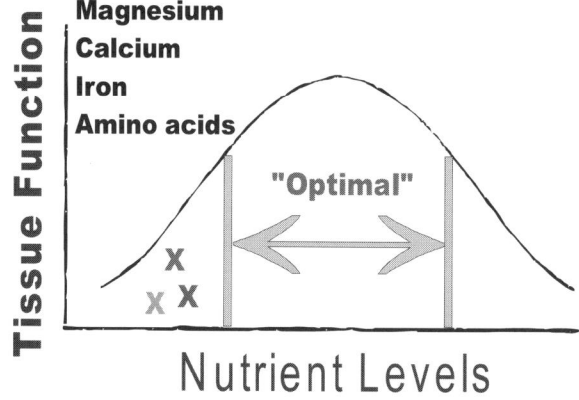

Tissue Function

Magnesium
Calcium
Iron
Amino acids

"Optimal"

X
X X

Nutrient Levels

Zinc and B6 in digestion

We can see that low Zinc will lead to poor digestion of proteins and dysbiosis.

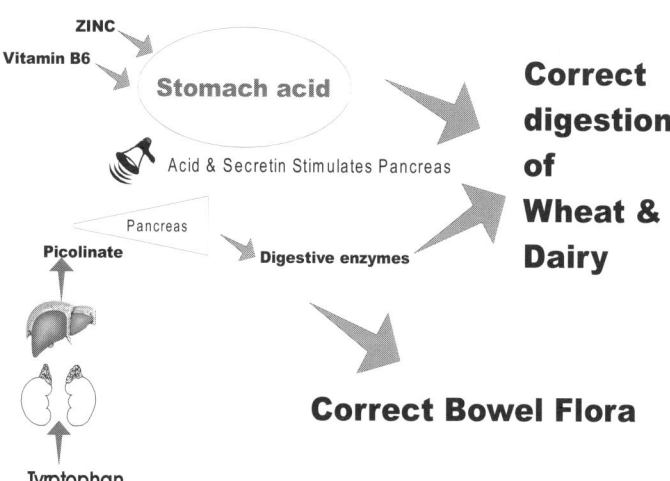

ZINC

Vitamin B6

Stomach acid

Acid & Secretin Stimulates Pancreas

Pancreas

Picolinate

Digestive enzymes

Tyrptophan

Correct digestion of Wheat & Dairy

Correct Bowel Flora

Intestinal Flora Balance

The knife-edge balance of bowel flora is very sensitive to intestinal Zinc levels.

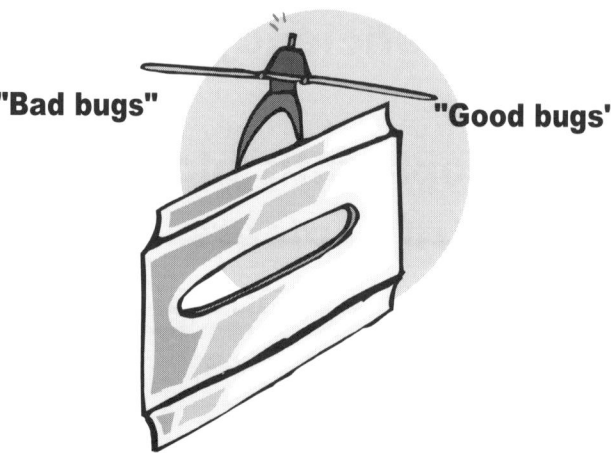

"Bad bugs"   "Good bugs"

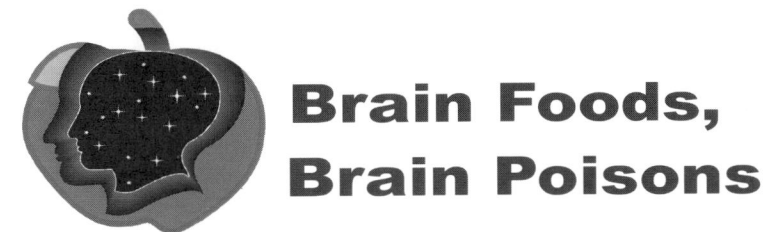

Brain Foods, Brain Poisons

So to summarise digestion, the process allows only inert nutrients into the body, but also keeps harmful things out of the body.

The Role of the digestive tract

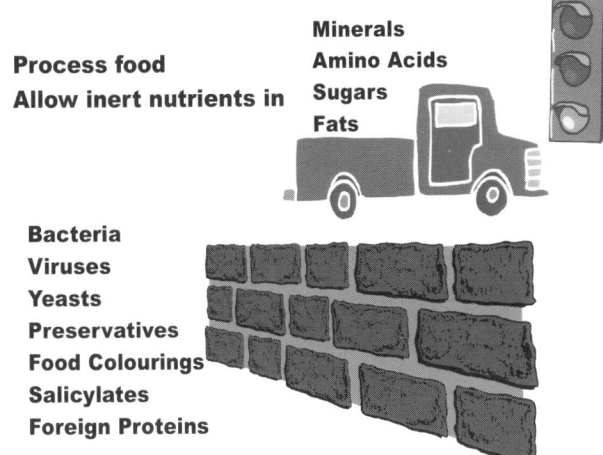

Process food
Allow inert nutrients in

Minerals
Amino Acids
Sugars
Fats

Bacteria
Viruses
Yeasts
Preservatives
Food Colourings
Salicylates
Foreign Proteins

Poor

Digestion

Poor digestion is a common finding in Autism.

Generation of antigliadin AB's

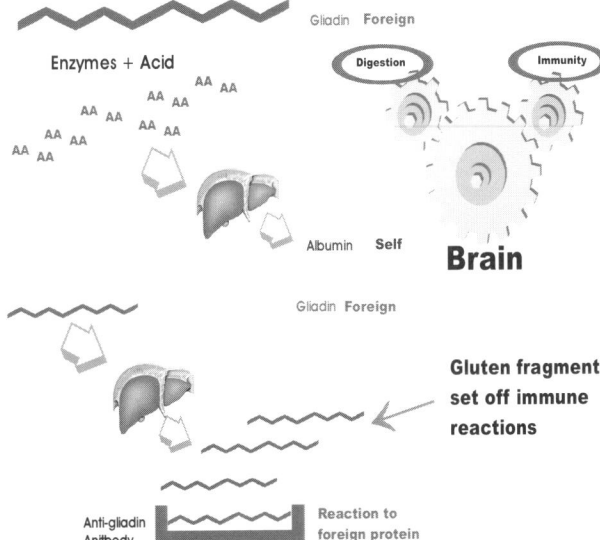

Gliadin Foreign

Enzymes + Acid

AA AA AA
AA AA AA AA
AA AA AA AA
AA AA
AA AA

Digestion   Immunity

Albumin   Self   **Brain**

Gliadin Foreign

**Gluten fragments
set off immune
reactions**

Anti-gliadin
Anitbody

Reaction to
foreign protein

The process of digestion is really converting foreign to self. Take a building apart, transport the bricks and use them for paving. Same bricks, different structure. If stomach acid is low, we get incomplete dismantling of proteins. Such fragments will induce an immune reaction. The T-cells say "that's a funny virus, let's make an anti-gliadin (gluten) anti-body!"

Brain Foods, Brain Poisons

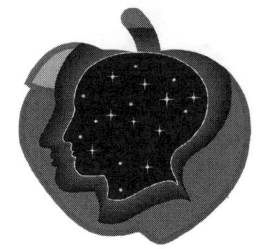

The same occurs for casein (especially A1 casein), hence the cross over with wheat and dairy. Just cutting them out only hides the problem. Fix the gut for a more permanent solution.

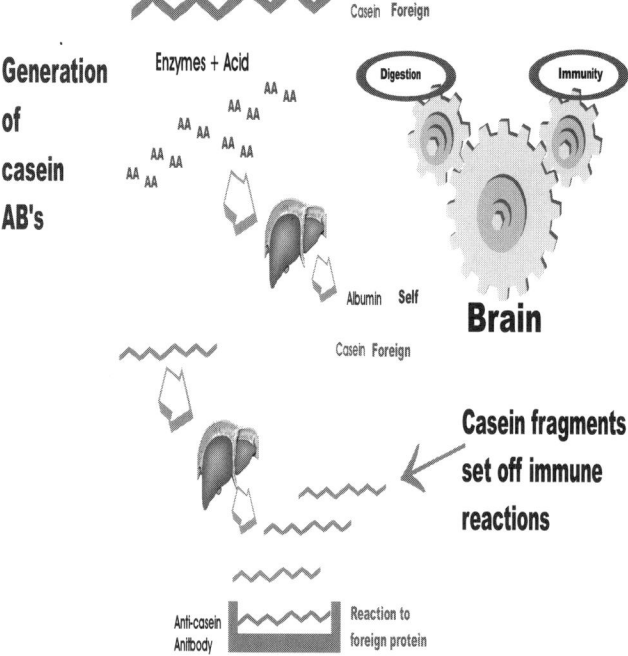

The final effect is that protein fragments (undigested peptides) will act like a spanner in the delicate cogs.

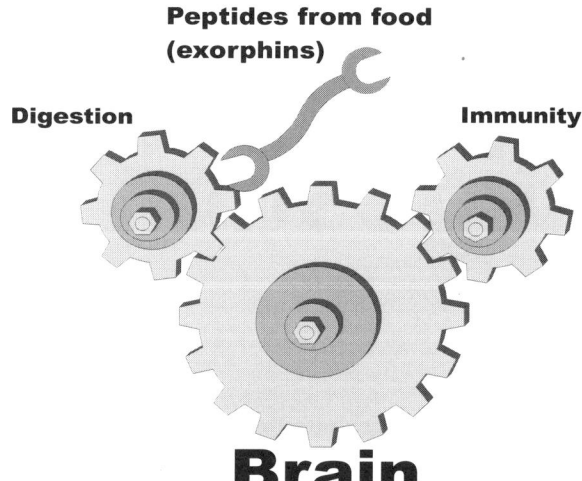

So in fact the reduction of symptoms by reducing wheat and dairy is explained by the presence of Zinc deficiency.

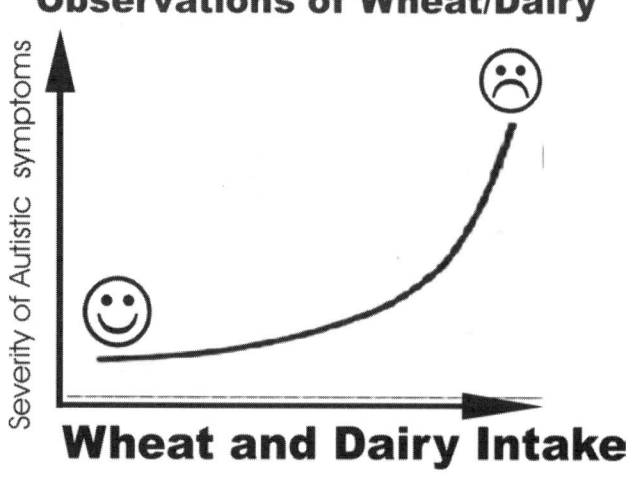

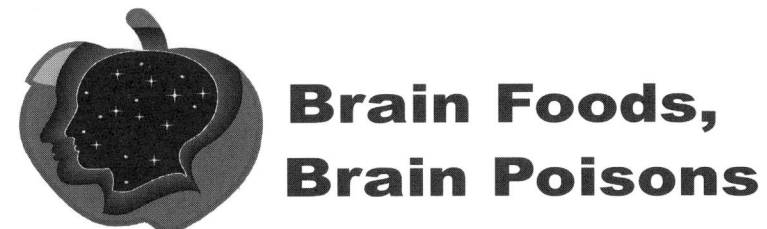

Brain Foods, Brain Poisons

Digestion is like Bee-keeping

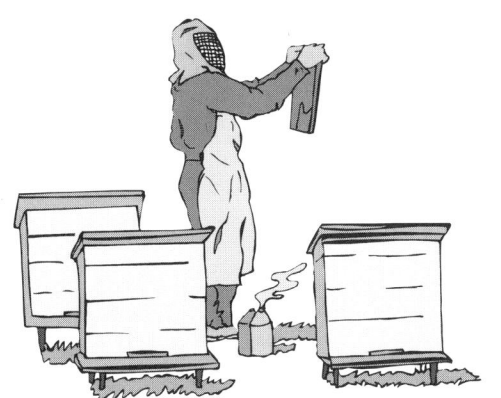

**You want the honey,
but you don't want to get stung!**

Digestion is like Bee-keeping. Zinc helps you get the Honey and prevents you from being stung.

Metabolic observations in Autism

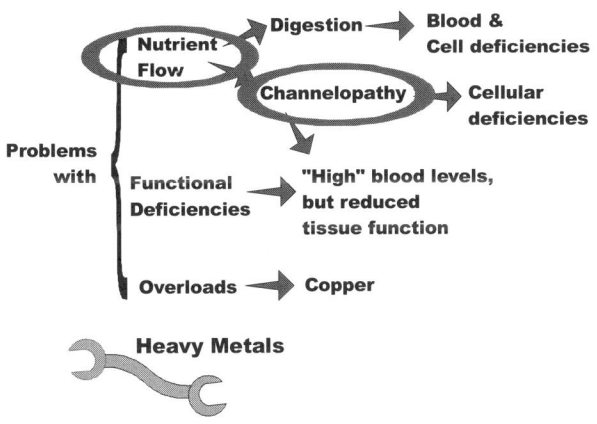

The next metabolic observation concerns low cellular levels of nutrients with apparently normal or high blood levels. This is the DOM definition of a Channelopathy (See extra notes at the end of this lecture).

2] Poor tissue uptake (Channelopathy)

BLOOD

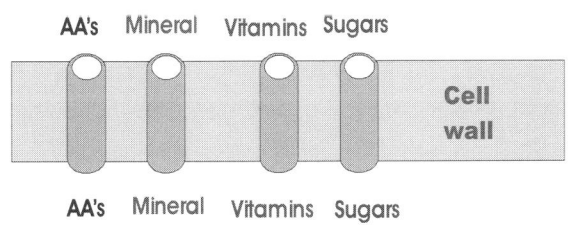

Cells

Transport of inert things from the gut continues on to the cells where "channels" allow the nutrient flow to continue. There is mounting evidence that dysfunctions of these channels are common and that these dysfunctions cause detectable human illnesses.

Brain Foods, Brain Poisons

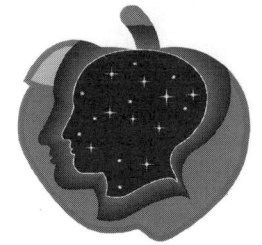

The two edged sword is that channels not only allow nutrients in, but they facilitate toxins to come out. This is important when we treat patients with such problems because we don't want to "destabilise" them too quickly.

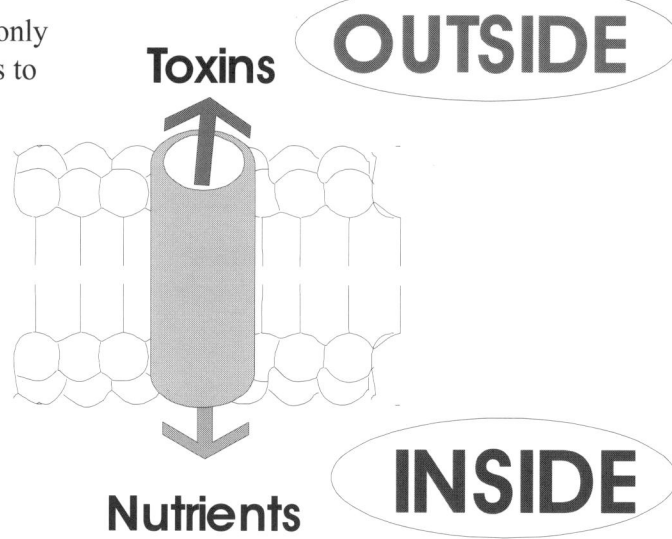

Some channels have a "hinged-pincer" structure like this Magnesium dependent Potassium channel. The membrane lipids (Essential Fatty Acids) at the edge of such channels need to be "flexible enough" to bend or compress when the channel is in operation. Hence the importance of EFA's in Channelopathies.

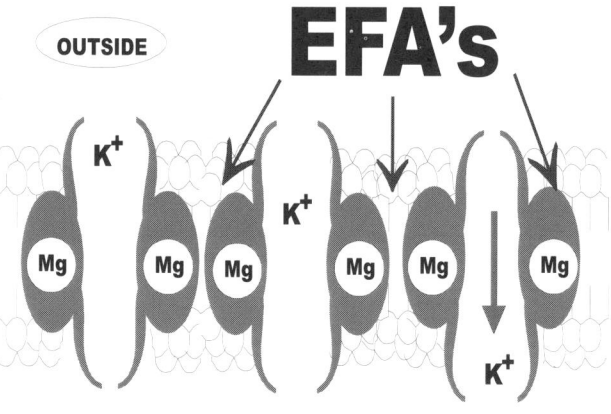

Effect of Mercury

Mercury is one of the "archetypal" channel blockers.

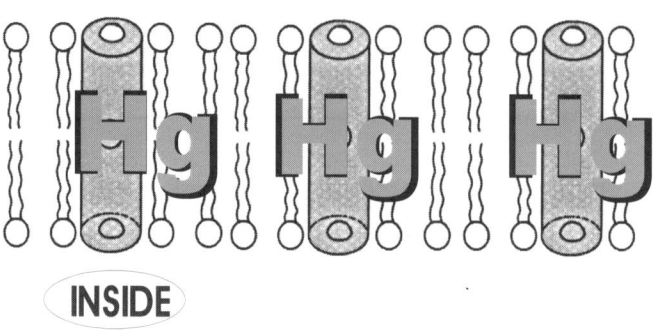

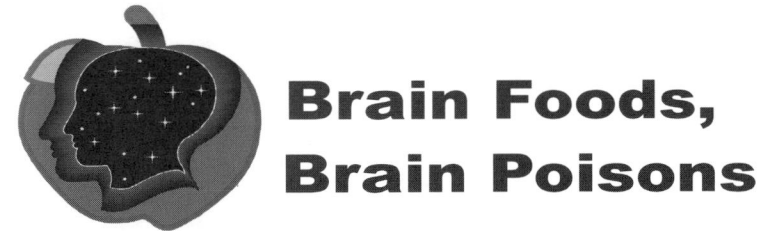

Brain Foods, Brain Poisons

Cellular deficiency

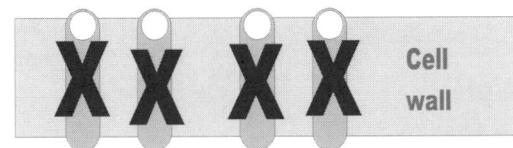

Vitamins Vitamins
Vitamins Vitamins
BLOOD Vitamins Vitamins
Vitamins Vitamins

X X X X   Cell wall

Cells

The effect of any Channel blocker is that nutrients cannot traverse cell membranes easily, and higher blood levels may be needed to "force" the movement via diffusion. This observation means that the "normal range" may not be the "optimum range" for patients with Channelopathies. Certainly a difficult concept for doctors and politically embarrassing since Doctors are criticised by the Health Insurance Commission (and Medical Boards) if the majority of their test come back in the "normal" range. Some have even been "struck off" for this.

Metabolic observations in Autism

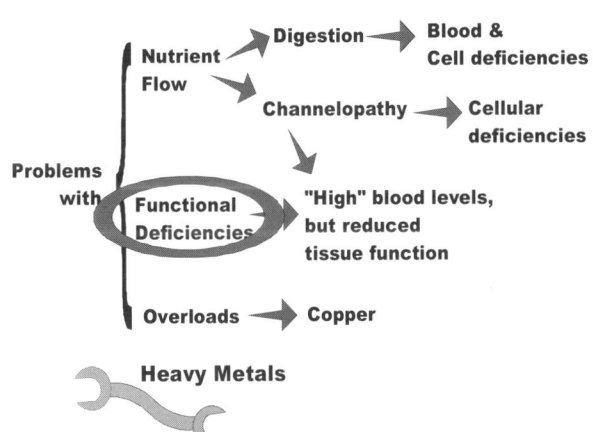

The next observation is that Nutrients may be present but disabled, creating so-called "functional" deficiencies. This may also lead to high blood levels because feedback mechanisms for transport rely on "activated" forms.

Nutrient utilisation

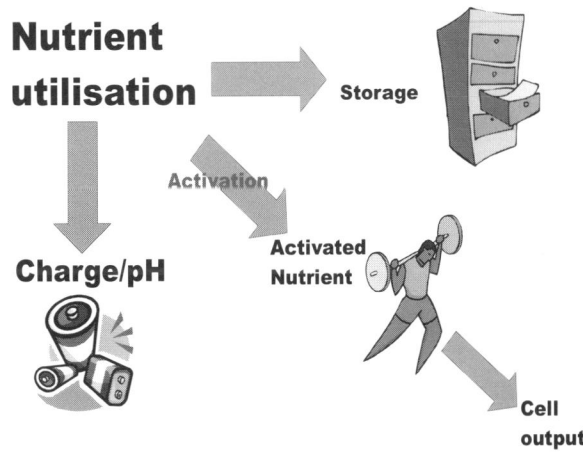

When nutrients enter the cells, they may wind up in several places. Firstly they may be stored. Secondly they may undergo activation into the final cofactor, which is used in enzymes, and thirdly they may be involved in charge or pH regulation.

Brain Foods, Brain Poisons

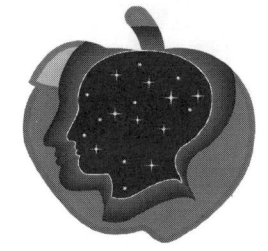

Toxin infiltration

Toxins infiltrate cells by "hitching a ride" with the nutrients (like a Trojan horse). They may get stored, they may block activation or they may disrupt charge/pH mechanisms.

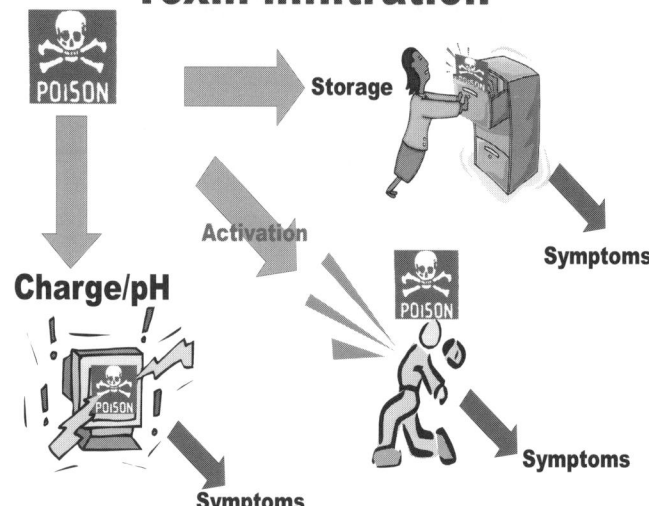

Metallic defence systems

In terms of storage, much is known about the metallic defence mechanisms (see chapter on "Lock up your Cations" at end of this section).

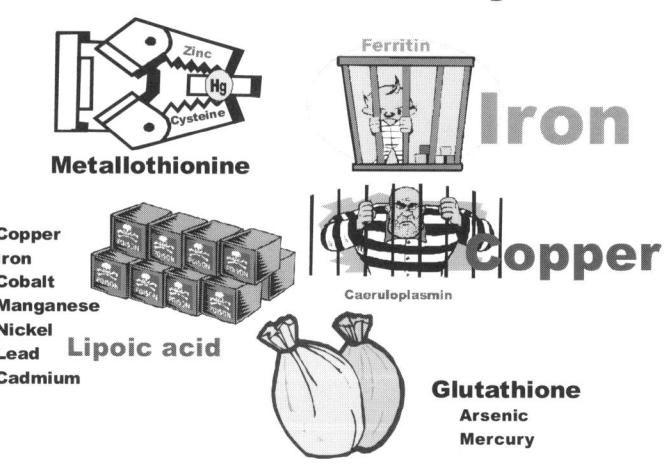

In the protective process of storing metals we create a stress on resources

The problem is that metal storage takes up resources.

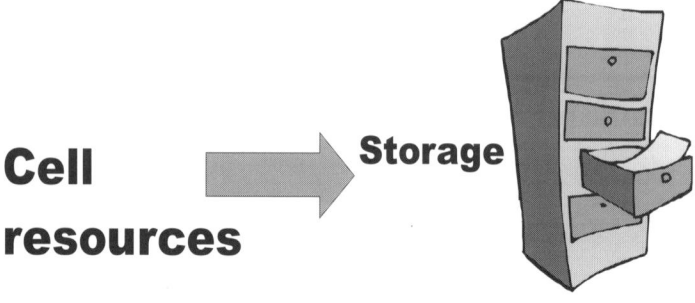

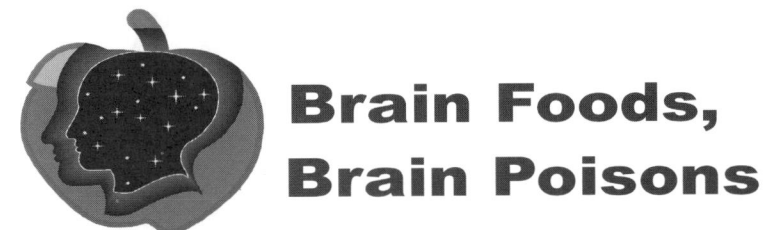

Brain Foods, Brain Poisons

Lipoic acid can Store Metals

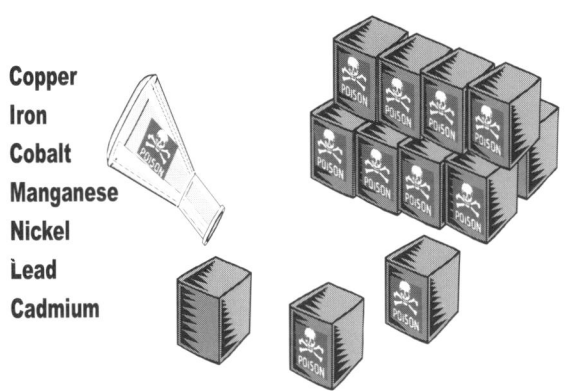

Copper
Iron
Cobalt
Manganese
Nickel
Lead
Cadmium

Resources like Lipoic Acid can certainly be used as "containment systems" for metals like Copper, Iron, Cobalt, Manganese, Nickel, Lead and Cadmium.

The Lipoic acid juggle

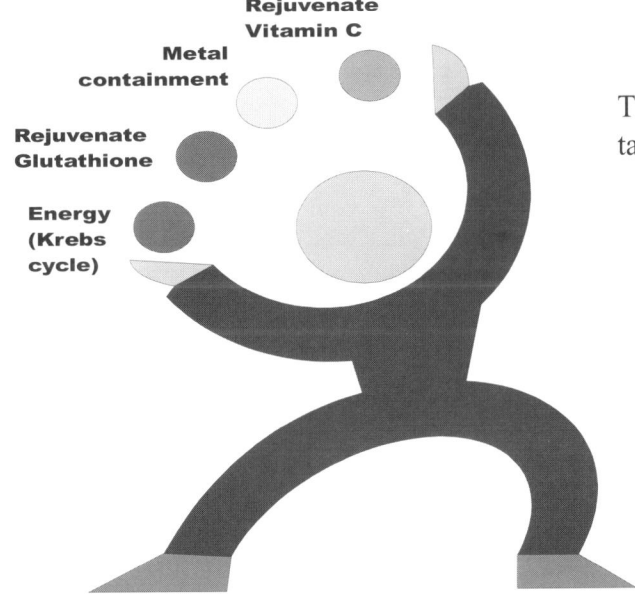

Rejuvenate
Vitamin C

Metal
containment

Rejuvenate
Glutathione

Energy
(Krebs
cycle)

The problem is that Lipoic acid is used for other tasks too. This creates the "Lipoic Acid Juggle"

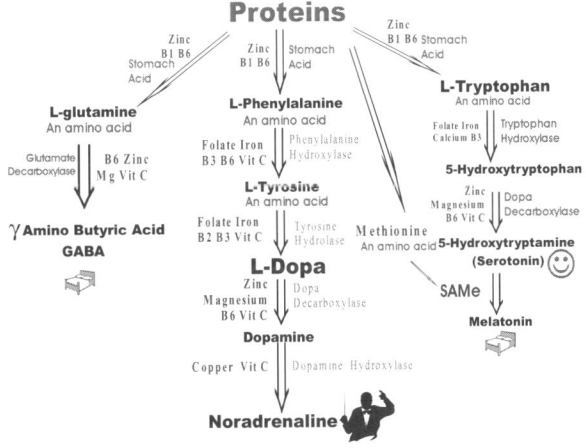

One of the tasks of Lipoic acid is regenerating Vitamin C. The Noradrenaline synthesis pathway needs Vitamin C in 4 consecutive steps. So Lipoic Acid levels will affect the function of Vitamin C and the efficiency of this pathway even though Lipoic acid is not a cofactor as such.

Brain Foods, Brain Poisons

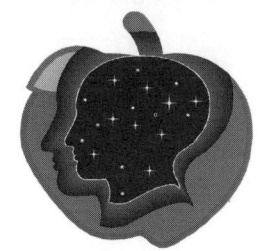

Why do we need Glutathione?

Metallic defence systems

In terms of Metallic defence, many of these containment systems are part of a "Juggle"

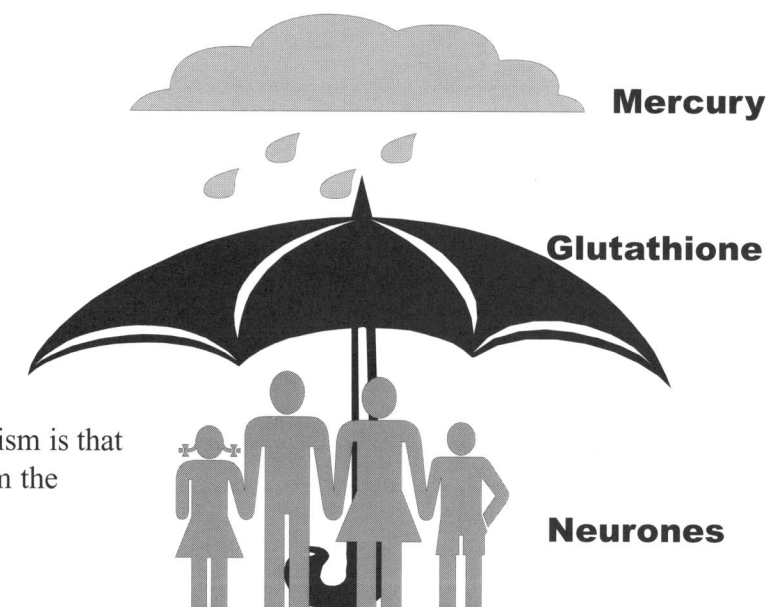

The relevance of glutathione in Autism is that Glutathione protects brain cells from the damaging effects of mercury.

Hair Mercury in Autism

The observation that severe Autistics may not be able to excrete Mercury has been postulated to explain the TMA findings.

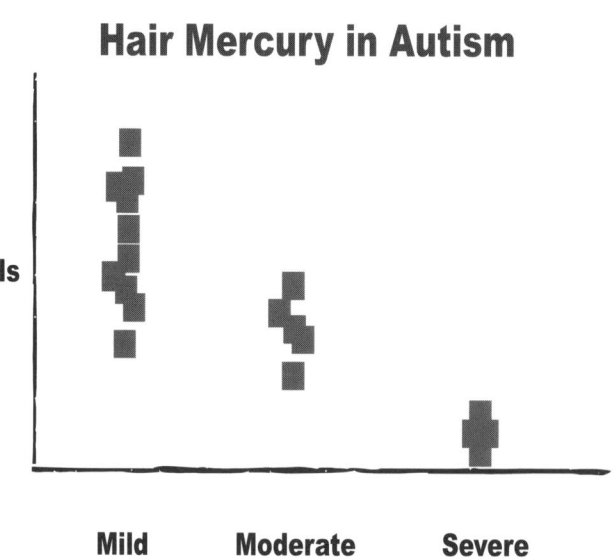

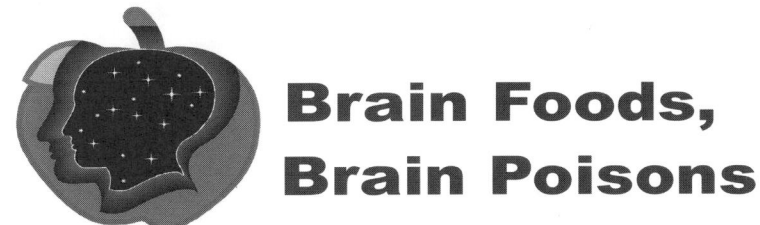

Brain Foods, Brain Poisons

The Glutathione juggle

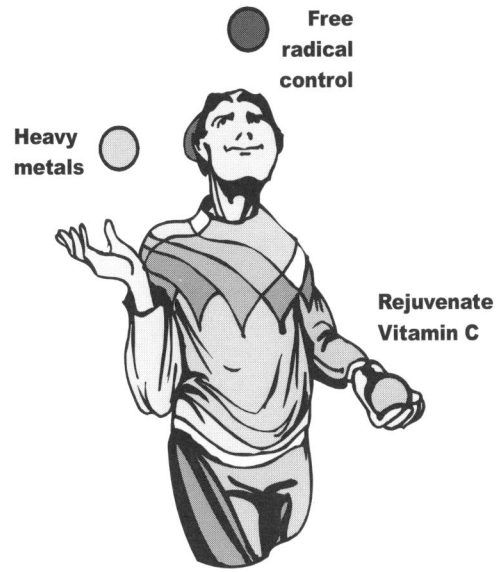

Free radical control

Heavy metals

Rejuvenate Vitamin C

We can see that there is a "Glutathione Juggle" too. Is it possible that the symptoms of Autism are due the <u>reason</u> that Mercury is retained, rather than the Mercury per se?

Glutathione

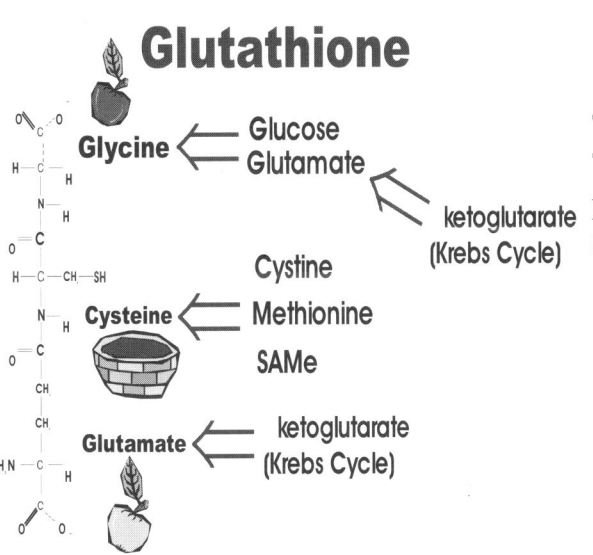

Glycine ← Glucose
Glutamate

ketoglutarate (Krebs Cycle)

Cystine
Cysteine ← Methionine
SAMe

Glutamate ← ketoglutarate (Krebs Cycle)

Think of Glutathione as 3 parts of a fruit basket. The basket is the Amino Acid Cysteine. The provision of this Amino Acid is the rate-limiting step in making Glutathione.

The brain needs glutathione

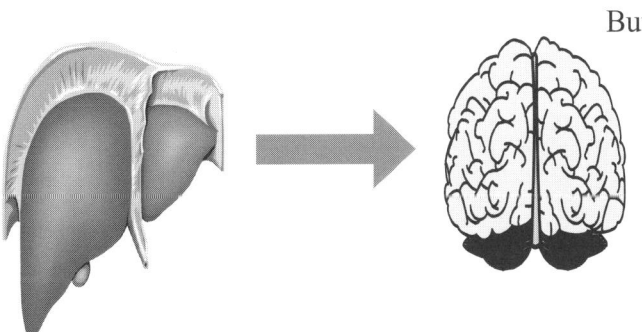

But how does the Brain get its glutathione?

The Liver sends some

Brain Foods, Brain Poisons

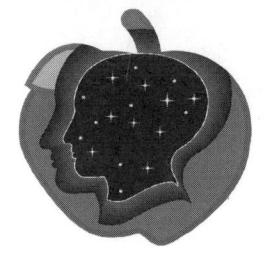

Liver

It's provided by the Liver in a very complex long-winded mechanism, which starts in the liver, moves to the blood, then to the Glial (Nanny) cells then to the space between the Glial cells and the Nerves, then into the Nerves.

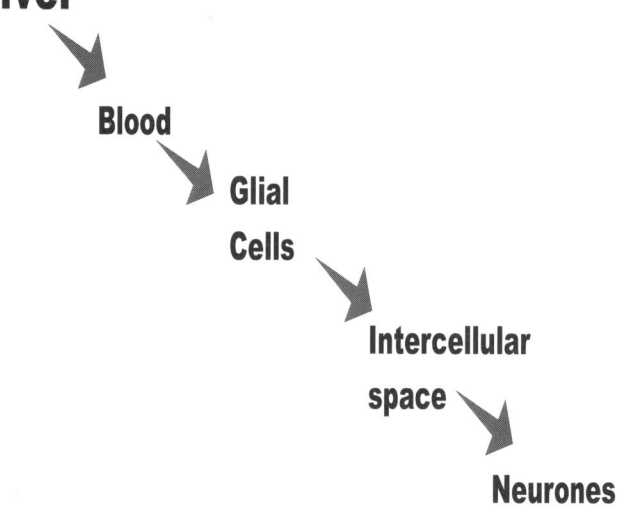

Liver

→ **Blood**

→ **Glial Cells**

→ **Intercellular space**

→ **Neurones**

In the liver

The Liver makes the basket (glutathione) in good faith.

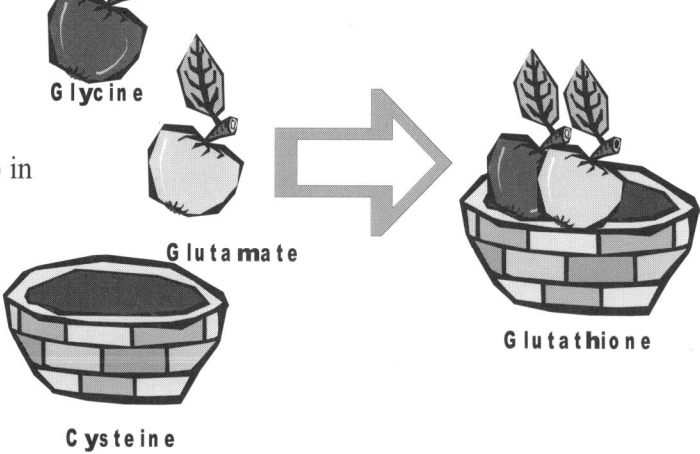

Glycine

Glutamate

Cysteine

Glutathione

In the bloodstream

It gently puts the basket into the bloodstream. But immediately the Enzyme Gamma-glutamyl transferase (the famous GGT) steps in. "Sorry, but you can't travel together. I'm splitting you up!"

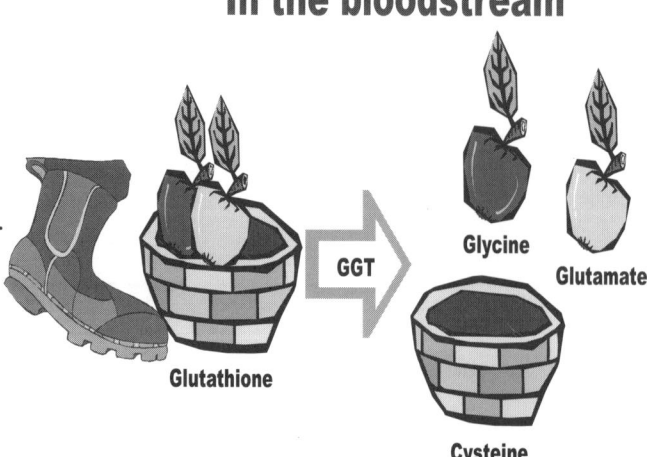

Glutathione

GGT

Glycine

Glutamate

Cysteine

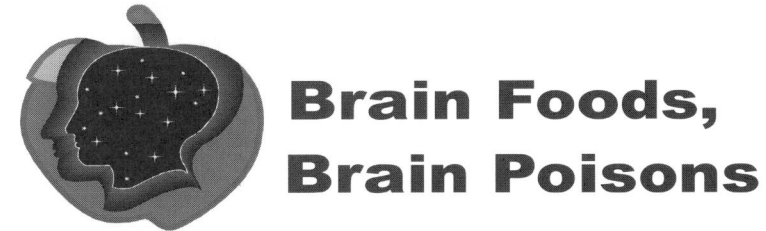

Brain Foods, Brain Poisons

In the bloodstream

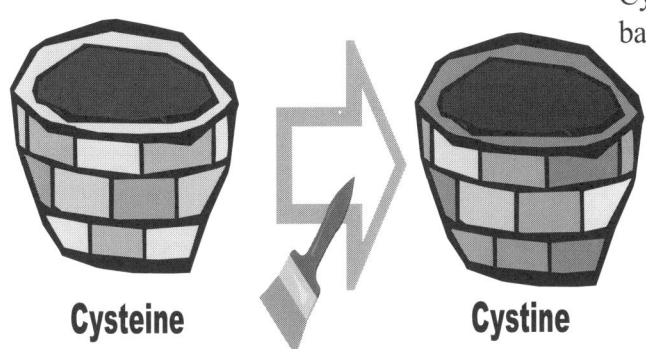

Cysteine   **Cystine**

Furthermore the blood doesn't like to transport Cysteine and converts to Cystine. " We like the basket, but we don't like the colour".

In the Glial Cell

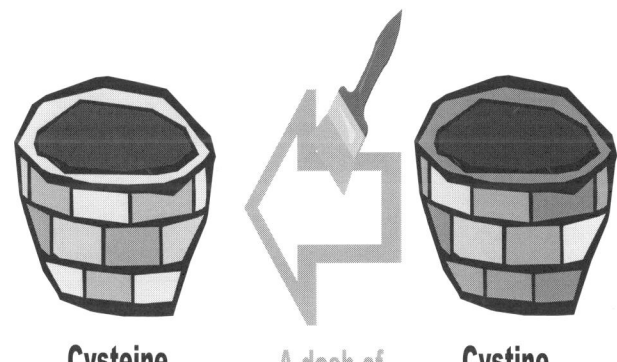

Cysteine   A dash of   **Cystine**
                 Lipoic acid

The Glial cell takes up the Cystine and changes it into Cysteine by using Lipoic acid. "We prefer the basket in the other colour"

In the Glial Cell

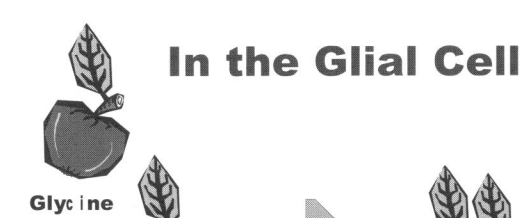
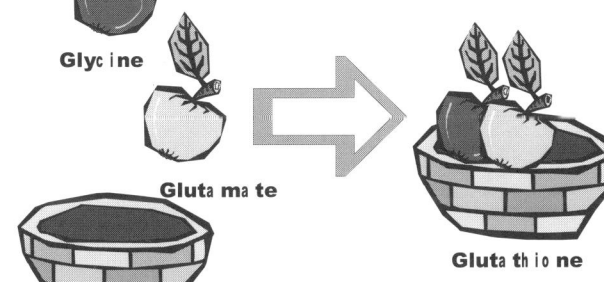

Glyc i ne

Gluta ma te

Cys tei ne

Gluta th io ne

The Glial cell reconstructs the fruit basket again.

Brain Foods, Brain Poisons

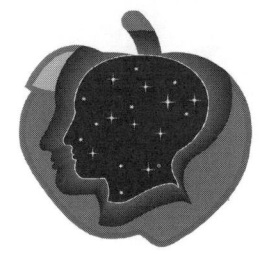

In the intracellular space

And in good faith sends it out into the interstitial space.

But again Gamma-Glutamyl transferase (GGT) says, "Sorry, but you can't travel together. I'm splitting you up!"

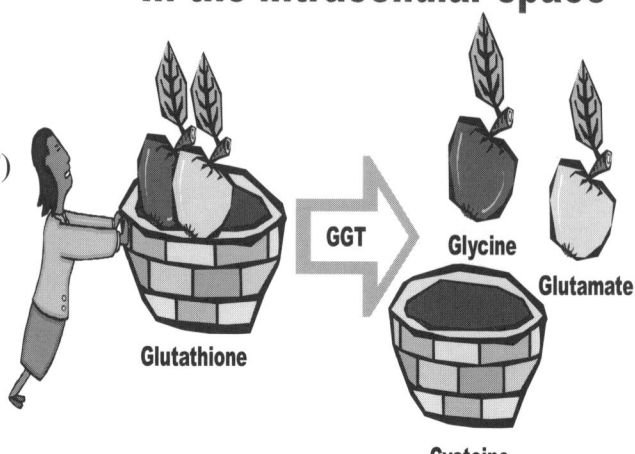

Finally in the neuron

Finally, the Nerve cells get the Cysteine (the only original component from the liver) and reconstruct the basket with some spare fruit. Wow, what a journey! Practitioners who give Glutathione orally or intravenously, must wonder what really happens after the patient gets it!

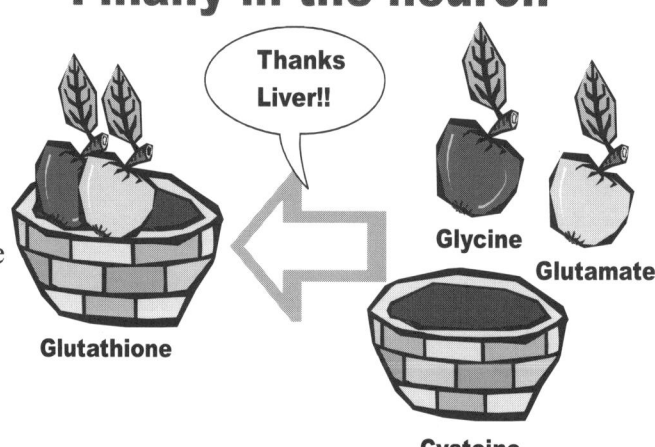

Metallic defence systems

Getting back to the metal defence systems, the most famous in Autism research is Metallothionine.

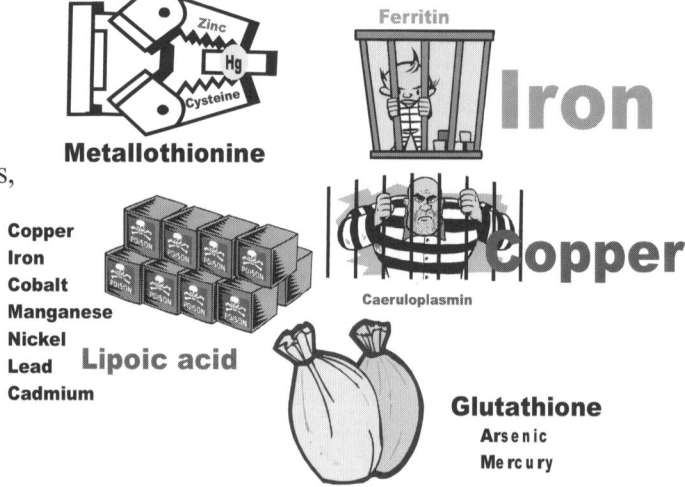

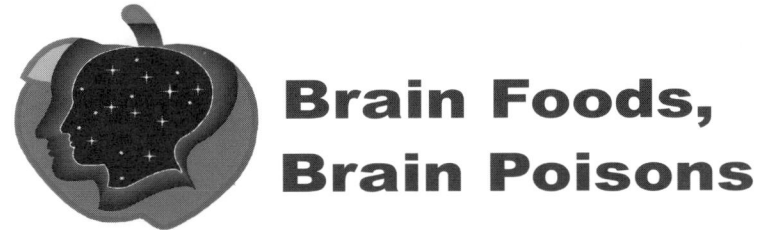

Brain Foods, Brain Poisons

The process of mercury excretion

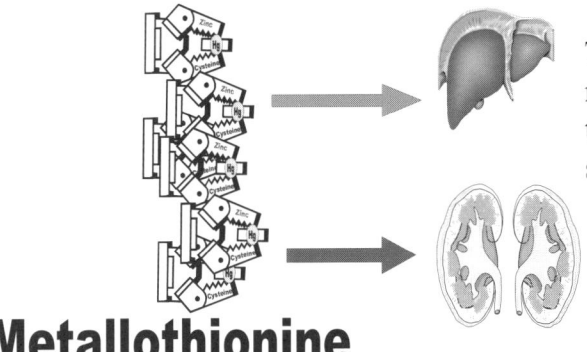

Metallothionine

The process of Mercury (and indeed Cadmium) removal is by the "locking up" of these metals in the pincer created by Zinc and Cysteine and sending it all off to the excretory organs.

Zinc and Sulphur "sacrificed"

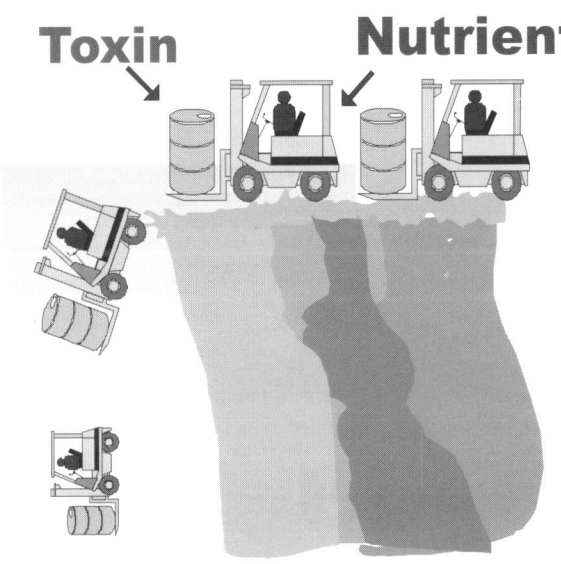

Toxin **Nutrient**

This means that Zinc and Cysteine are "sacrificed" in order to get rid of mercury and Cadmium.

Metallothionine Structure

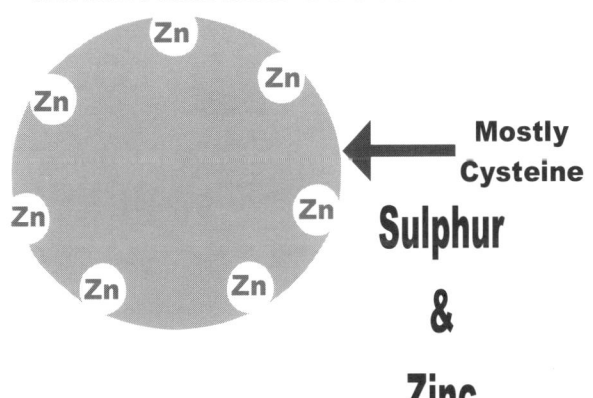

Zn Zn Zn Zn Zn Zn Zn

Mostly Cysteine

Sulphur & Zinc

Another way to visualise Metallothionine is to think of it as a big ball of sulphur and zinc.

Brain Foods, Brain Poisons

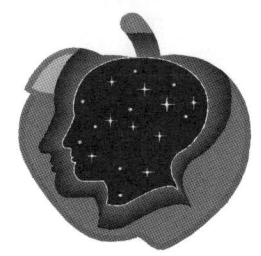

Functions of Metallothionine

It appears in several places in the body, where it has interesting functions. Most of it (two-thirds) is in the intestine.

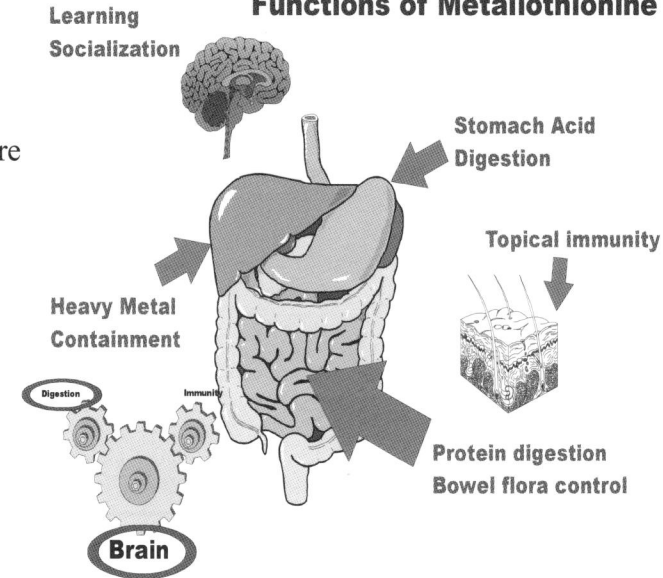

Learning
Socialization

Stomach Acid
Digestion

Topical immunity

Heavy Metal
Containment

Protein digestion
Bowel flora control

Digestion

Immunity

Brain

The Zinc juggle

But again storage of metals places stress on resources and so we have a "Zinc Juggle" too.

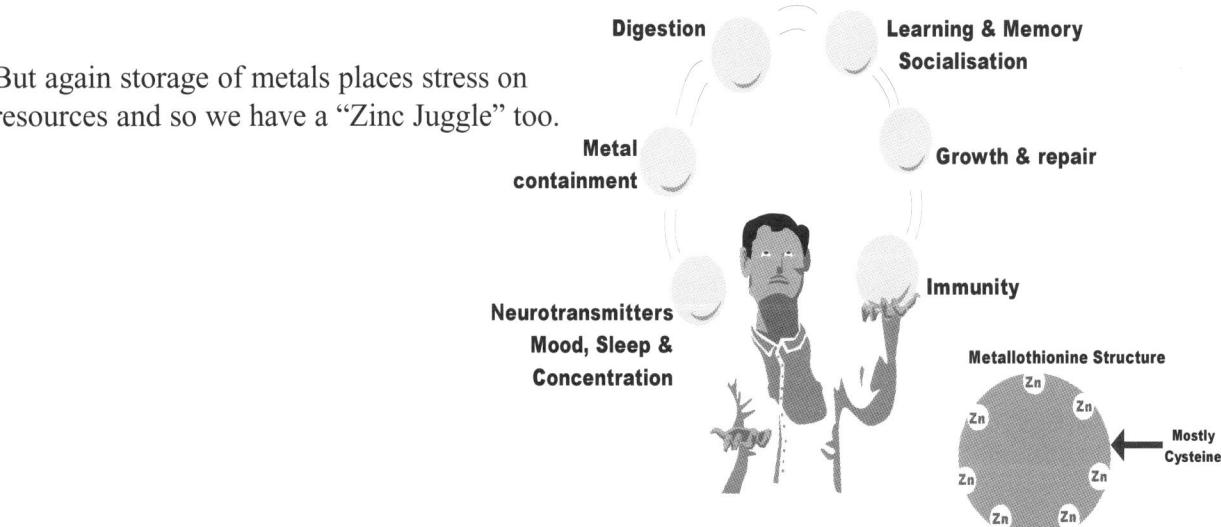

Digestion

Learning & Memory
Socialisation

Metal
containment

Growth & repair

Immunity

Neurotransmitters
Mood, Sleep &
Concentration

Metallothionine Structure

Zn Zn Zn Zn Zn Zn

Mostly
Cysteine

Metallic defence systems

But 3 of these metallic defence systems need Cysteine to make them.

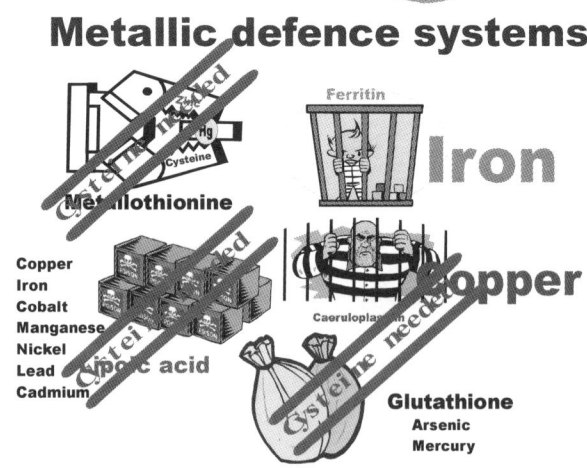

Ferritin

Iron

Metallothionine

Copper
Iron
Cobalt
Manganese
Nickel
Lead
Cadmium

Caeruloplasmin

Copper

Lipoic acid

Glutathione
Arsenic
Mercury

26

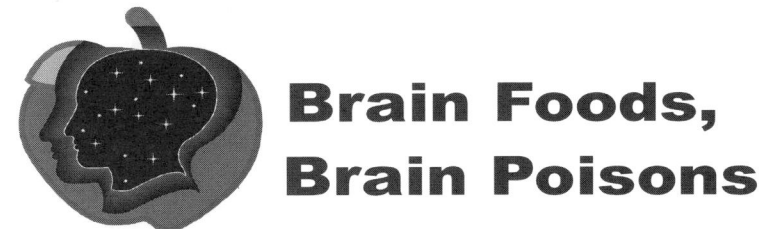

Brain Foods, Brain Poisons

The Cysteine juggle

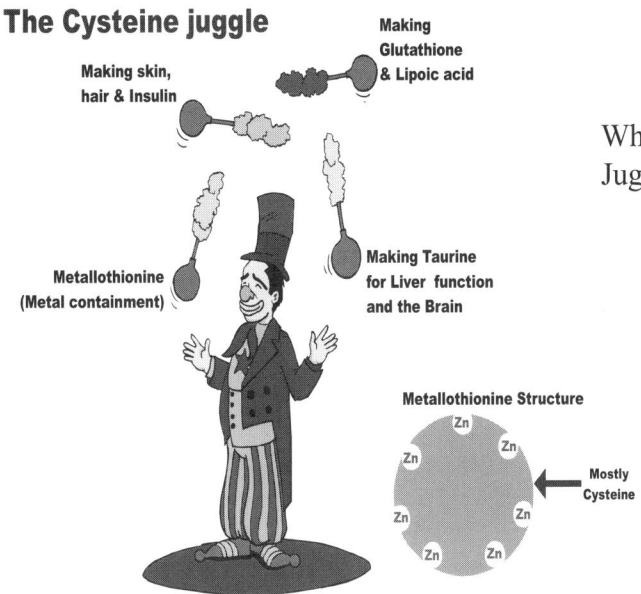

Making Glutathione & Lipoic acid

Making skin, hair & Insulin

Metallothionine (Metal containment)

Making Taurine for Liver function and the Brain

Metallothionine Structure

Zn Zn Zn Zn Zn Zn

← Mostly Cysteine

Which, you guessed it, creates the "Cysteine Juggle".

The resource juggle

Metals like Zinc & Copper

Cysteine

Energy

Glutathione

Lipoic acid

Vitamin C

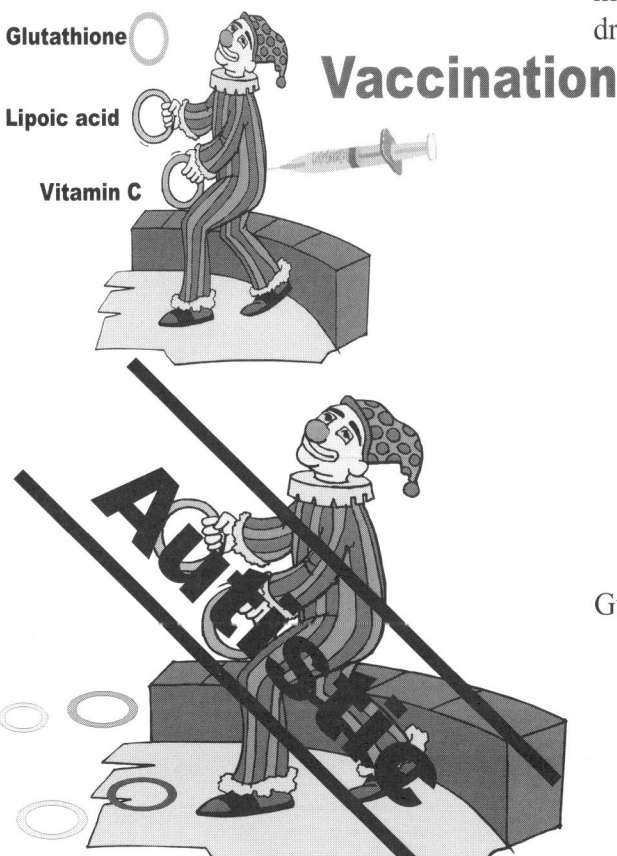

Vaccination

So what if we are trying to juggle all these metabolic resources and something makes us drop the whole lot?

Guess what label this condition would get?

Brain Foods, Brain Poisons

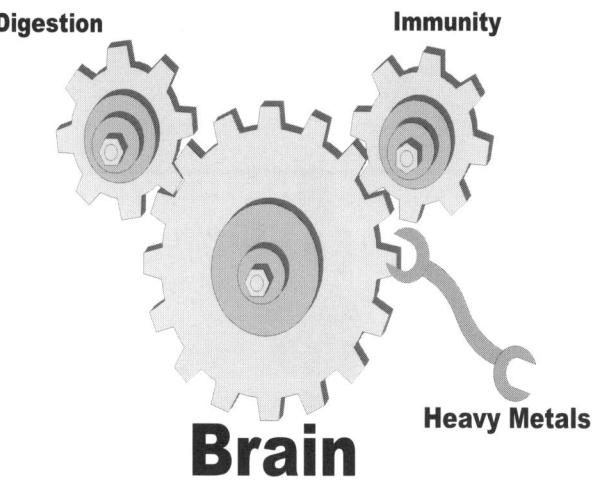

Next we look at the spanner of heavy metals that affect the integration of the cogs.

Toxins in Autism

The finger of blame has been pointed squarely at Mercury in Autism.

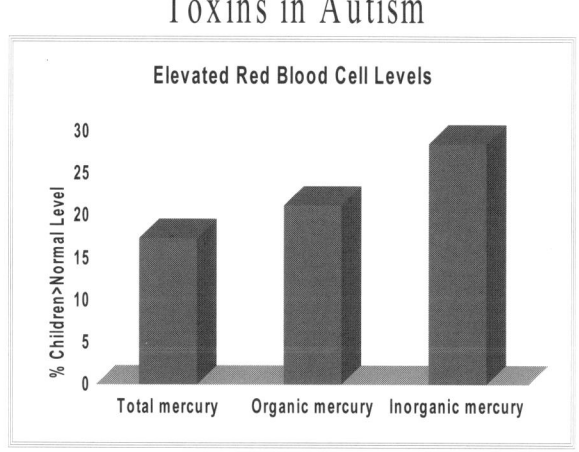

However, an interesting observation is made. Mercury is present in many chronic illnesses, but seems that the more severe the Autism, the harder it is to get rid of mercury.

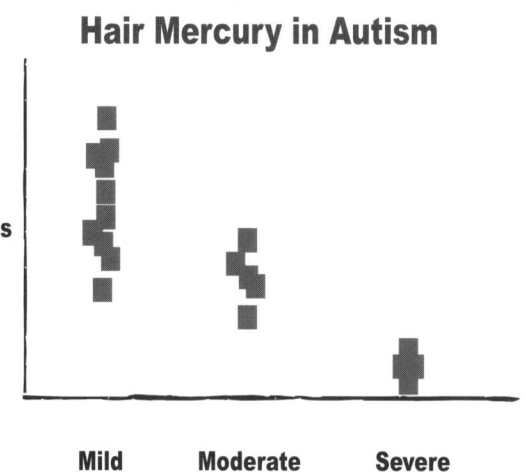

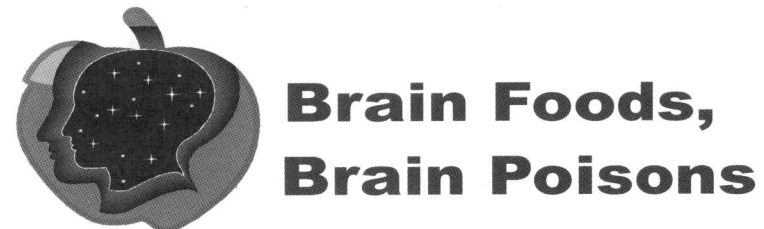

Brain Foods, Brain Poisons

Delayed Mercury excretion Model 1

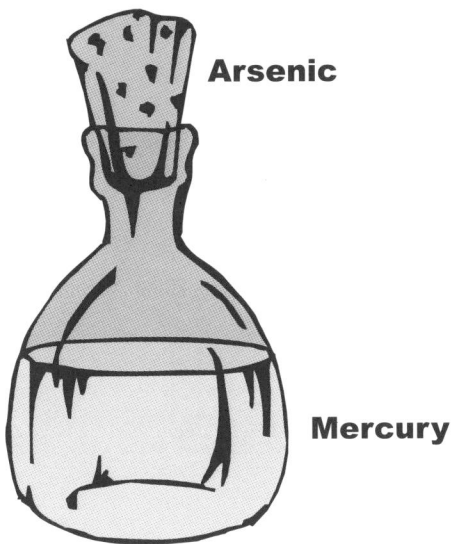

Arsenic

Mercury

There are many theories. Perhaps Arsenic acts like a cork that stops Mercury from getting out? It is true that many chelating practitioners often find Arsenic is the first toxin to vacate. They find that Mercury excretion may be delayed because of it; that DMSA /DMPS provocations may not show Mercury in the first instance.

Delayed Mercury excretion Model 2

Q. Do I have all the tools and safety equipment to do this?

Perhaps the body does not have all the gear to perform the excretion safely, and that is why Mercury may be retained inappropriately?

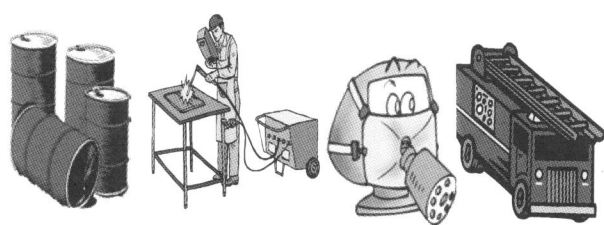

Delayed Mercury excretion Model 3

Funnel analogy for toxins

Mercury   Arsenic

Copper   Lead

Could it be that in the "higher purpose" of things that these toxins have to share exit points from the body?

Brain Foods, Brain Poisons

Could it be that the order of priority might not be what the practitioner intended? That the metals "take a ticket" and this ticketing determines the order and rate of removal of things?

Delayed Mercury excretion Model 3

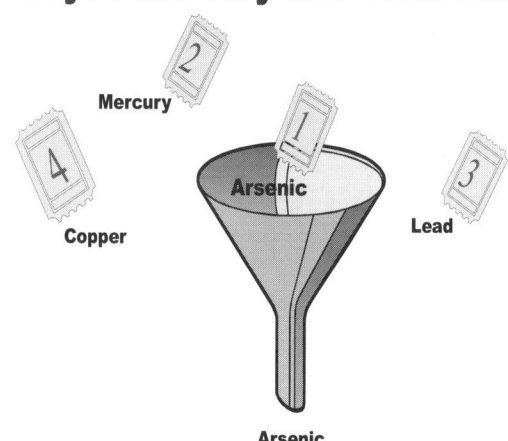

Anti-nutrients

Lead blocks Iron Calcium Molybdenum Manganese Chromium Sulphur Cobalt

Mercury blocks Zinc selenium iron sulphur cobalt transmembrane ion channels

But mercury is not the only toxin around. Perhaps it is important to consider all the toxins, not just one of them?

Cadmium blocks Zinc Magnesium Selenium Sulphur

Arsenic blocks Vit E selenium sulphur boron

Aluminium blocks Vit E Vit C Vit B1 Zinc Selenium Sodium Potassium Phosphorus

Antimony blocks Zinc Selenium

Perhaps the TMA's could be looked at thus. Imagine a card game like Gin Rummy or Poker. The nutrient elements are the cards you want to keep and the toxic elements are the cards you want to get rid of.

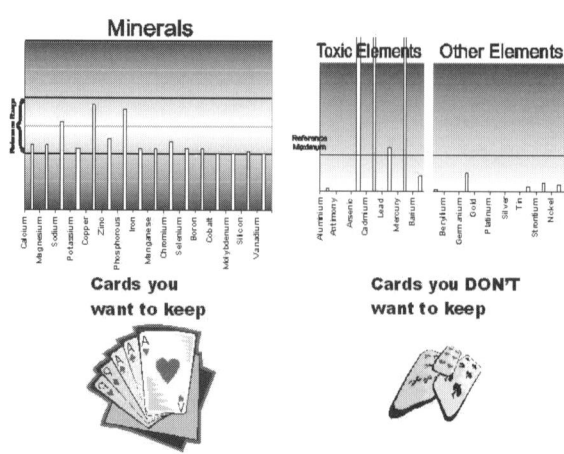

30

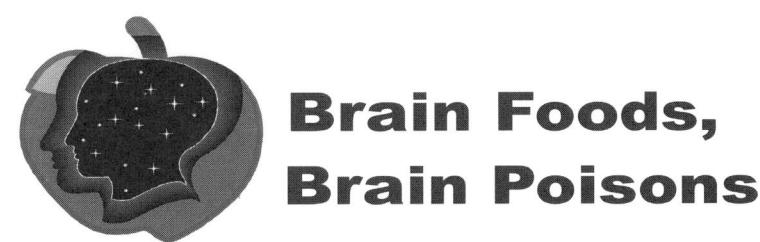

Brain Foods, Brain Poisons

Toxin defence

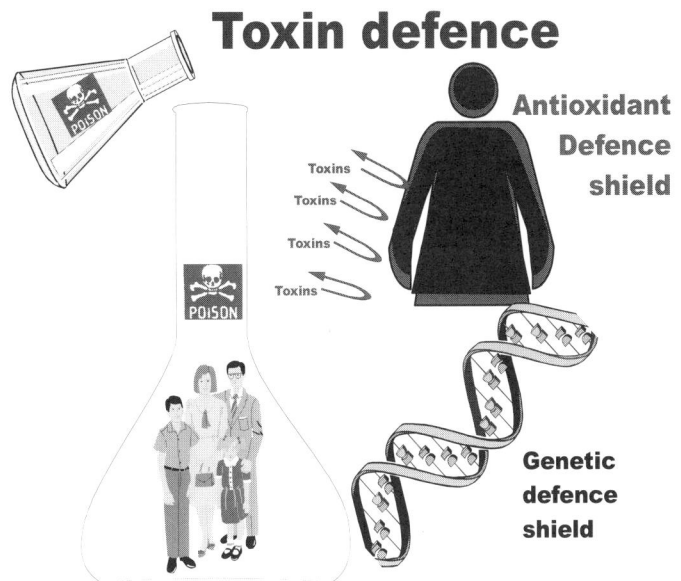

Antioxidant Defence shield

Toxins
Toxins
Toxins
Toxins

Genetic defence shield

So what about the combined effect of toxin exposure, Antioxidant defence and Genetic predisposition?

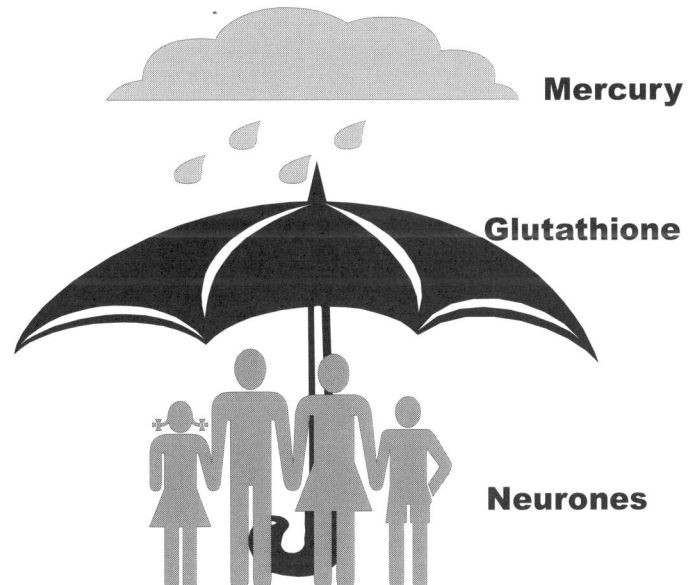

Mercury

Glutathione

Neurones

In order to understand this we need to know something of the protective systems like Glutathione.

Antioxidants

Metals	Vitamins
Zinc Copper Manganese Selenium Molybdenum	Vitamin A Vitamin C Vitamin E
Aminoacid derived Coenzyme Q10 Glutathione Lipioic acid	Bioflavonoids Beta carotene grapeseed extract pine bark extract lycopene quercetin rutin ,hesperidin

We know that Antioxidants help protect us from toxins.

Brain Foods, Brain Poisons

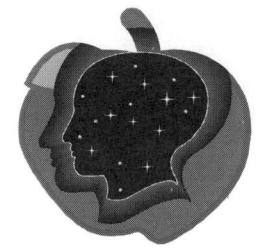

They are like the airbag in a car. They don't stop the crash, but they reduce the injuries from the crash.

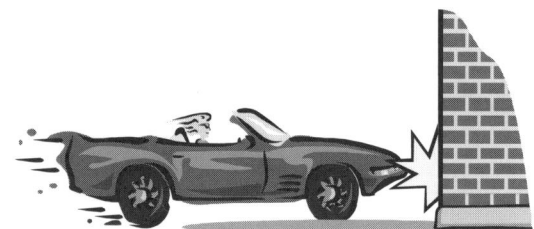

Antioxidant air-bag

Toxins "hitch a ride" with the nutrients

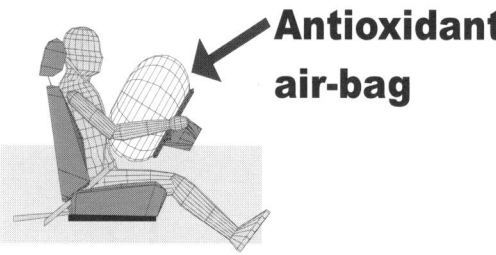

Cells

Environment

Environmental toxins "hitch a ride with nutrients". They get in through the food chain, for instance. The most notorious of these are from the "Zinc series" of the periodic table. They are Zinc, Cadmium and Mercury. See the article at the end on these metals.

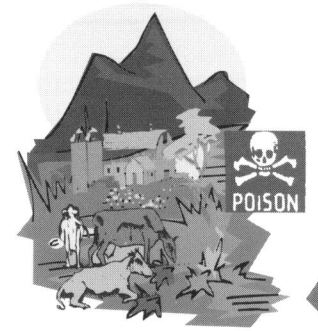

The "zinc series" of the periodic table

	30 Zn 65.37	
48 Cd 112.40	
80 Hg 200.59	

Plants will substitute Zinc Cadmium Mercury

Humans will substitute Zinc, Cadmium Mercury

Total Mercury Load

Does anyone add up the total environmental exposure?

Despite much being known about where Mercury comes from, very little attempt is made to add up the whole environmental exposure.

Vaccines **Fish & Seafood** **Amalgam Fillings** **Air Pollution**

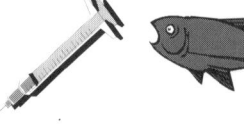
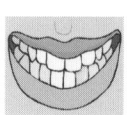
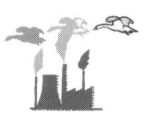

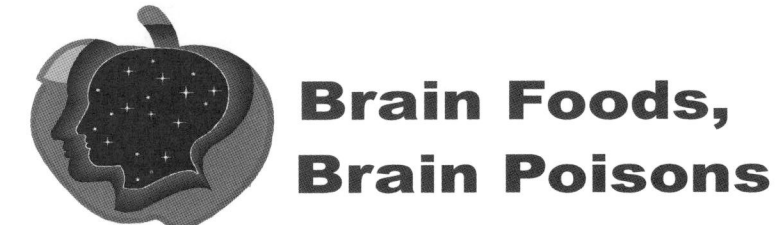

Brain Foods, Brain Poisons

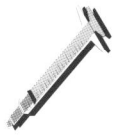

Total potential mercury load with full vaccination schedule using Thiomersal

273 micrograms

If we assess each contributor we can break down the addition. A full vaccination schedule with Thiomersol based vaccines could lead to a total mercury loading of 273 micrograms.

Fishing in Sydney

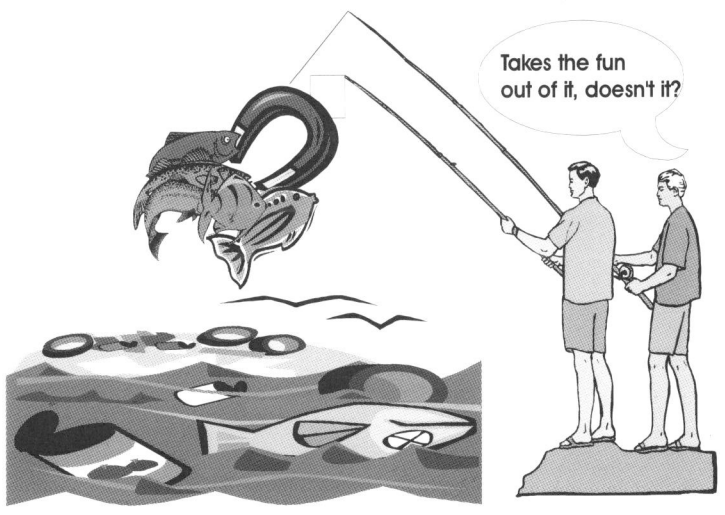

Takes the fun out of it, doesn't it?

Adapted from Zanetti's cartoon 1989

We are constantly being told to be careful of fish intake over time especially with women of childbearing age. This is a cartoon from a Sydney newspaper from 1989, when it was realised how high the heavy metals were in the local fish. But don't worry, FSANZ (Food Standards Australia and New Zealand) "is keeping an eye on things" for us.

Atmospheric Mercury pollution

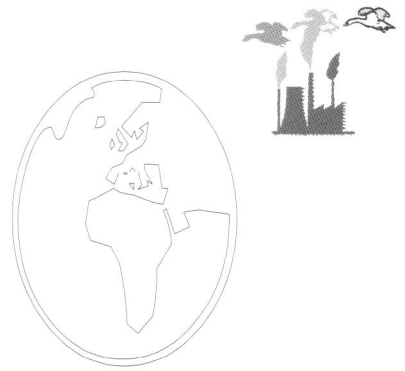

30 million tons per year globally

More worrisome is the fact that 30 million tons of Mercury is pumped into the atmosphere every year on this planet. Considering we worry about 273 micrograms, maybe we should worry about 30 million tons too?

Brain Foods, Brain Poisons

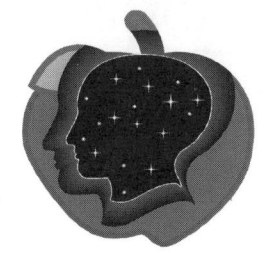

Optimistic Mercury Life Time Line

So we expect the total Mercury level to rise over a lifetime; each contributor adding to the "pot". The optimists would say that we have plenty of ability to cope with this load and we will never exceed the tolerable limit.

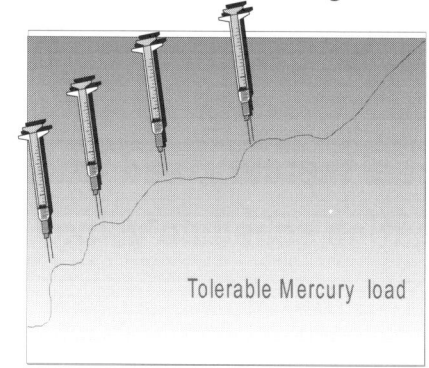

Rising background mercury levels
Fish
Pollution
Amalgams

Tolerable Mercury load

Time in years

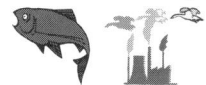 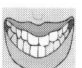

Real world Mercury Life Time Line

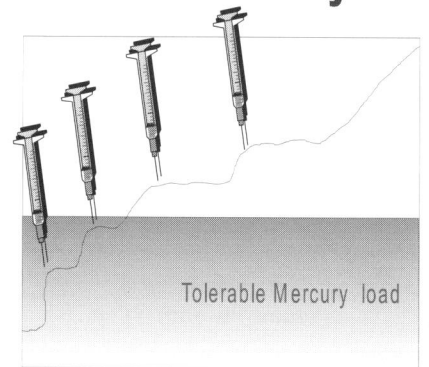

But what if they were wrong? What if we are already seeing that some individuals have exceeded this limit?

Rising background mercury levels
Fish
Pollution
Amalgams

Tolerable Mercury load

Time in years

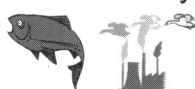

Total "Domestic" Mercury Load

On a population basis, at what point will we see the limit exceed in general? Have we already passed this point?

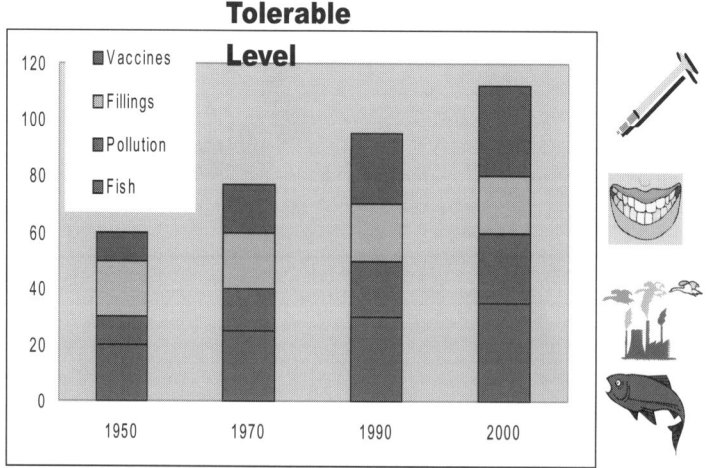

Maximum Tolerable Level

Legend: Vaccines, Fillings, Pollution, Fish

34

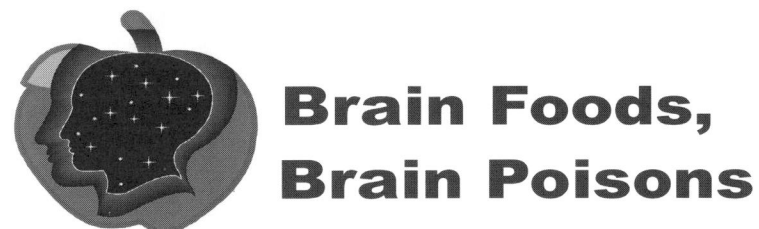

Brain Foods, Brain Poisons

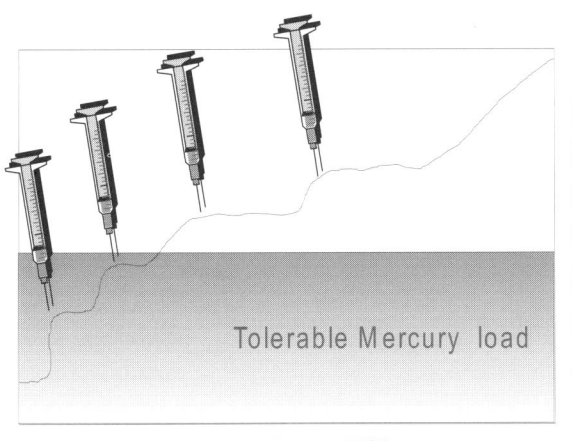

Rising background mercury levels
Fish
Pollution
Amalgams

Tolerable Mercury load

Scientific literature has implicated Mercury in Alzheimer's disease and Cardiovascular disease. The dementia that occurs in later life has certain symptoms that if "recreated in younger people, would get different labels from medicine. Could Autism and Alzheimer's be linked in this way?

DSMIV label at different ages

0-2	2-18	18-50	50 plus
Delayed milestones	ADD	Brain fog	Dementia

Pre-natal Mercury Time Line

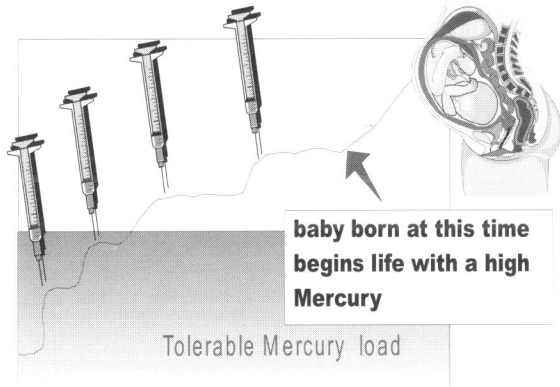

baby born at this time begins life with a high Mercury

Tolerable Mercury load

Time in years

The next concern is that if each generation's Mercury load is slightly higher, then at some point a baby will be born with an intolerable load from day 1.

Toxin infiltration & Defence

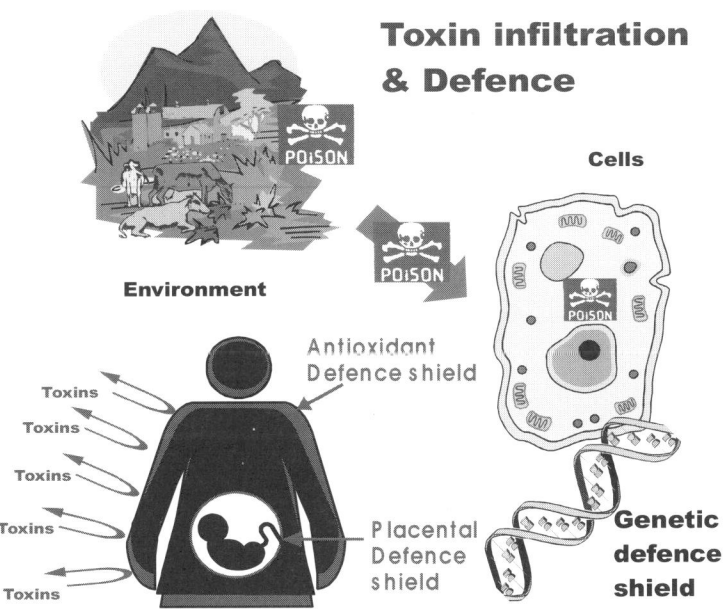

Cells

POISON

Environment

POISON

POISON

Toxins

Toxins

Toxins

Toxins

Toxins

Antioxidant Defence shield

Placental Defence shield

Genetic defence shield

This means that the Antioxidant defence system has to be up and running in the Mother (just like the leukaemia study showed) and that those genes may change the level of vulnerability.

Brain Foods, Brain Poisons

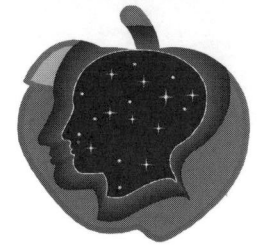

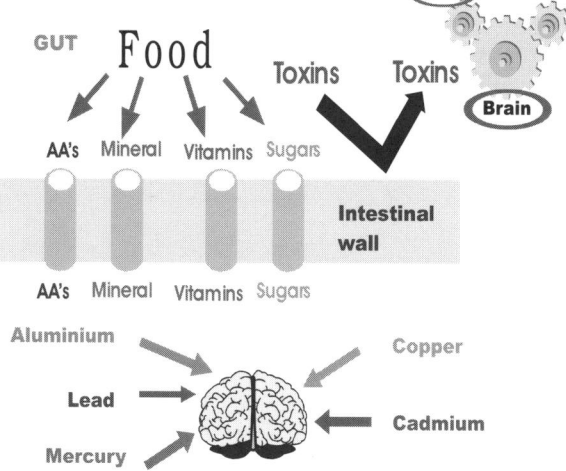

Toxins such as Mercury & Aluminium want to move to the brain. It is up to our digestive tract (including the liver) to prevent this. So digestion and brain function are linked in this way.

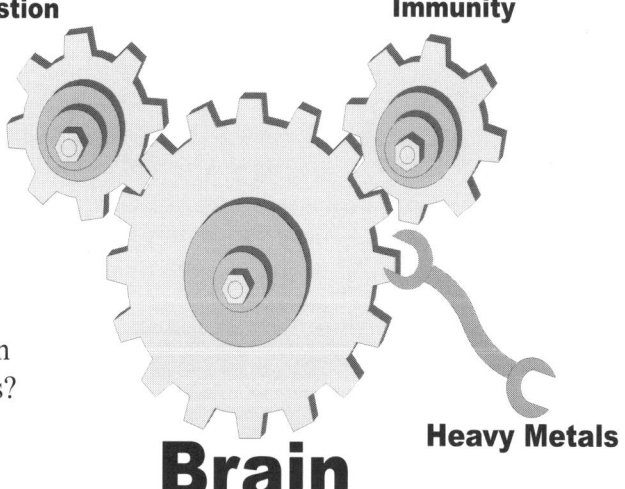

Hence the association of heavy metals and Autism. Could it be that the cause of Autism is actually the reason these metals can't be screened out from the intestinal tract, rather than the presence of these globally ubiquitous metals?

Metabolic observations in Autism

Moving on from heavy metals to Functional deficiencies.

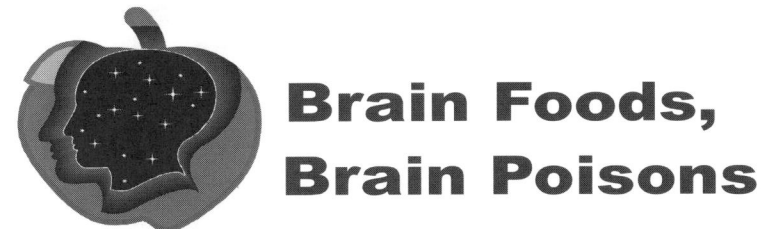

Brain Foods, Brain Poisons

Nutrient flow & Functional deficiencies

We find high levels of "ineffective nutrients" sometimes. Let's look at the mechanisms.

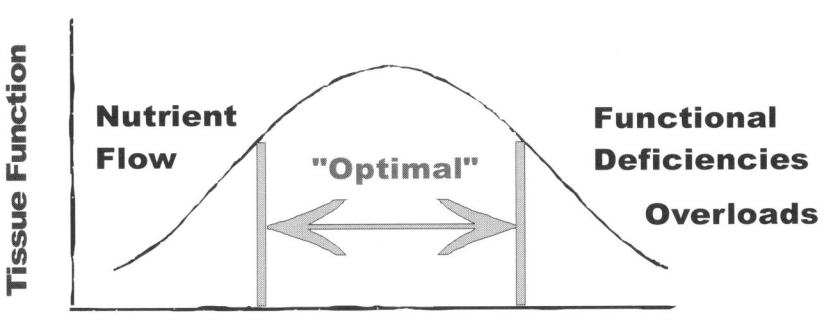

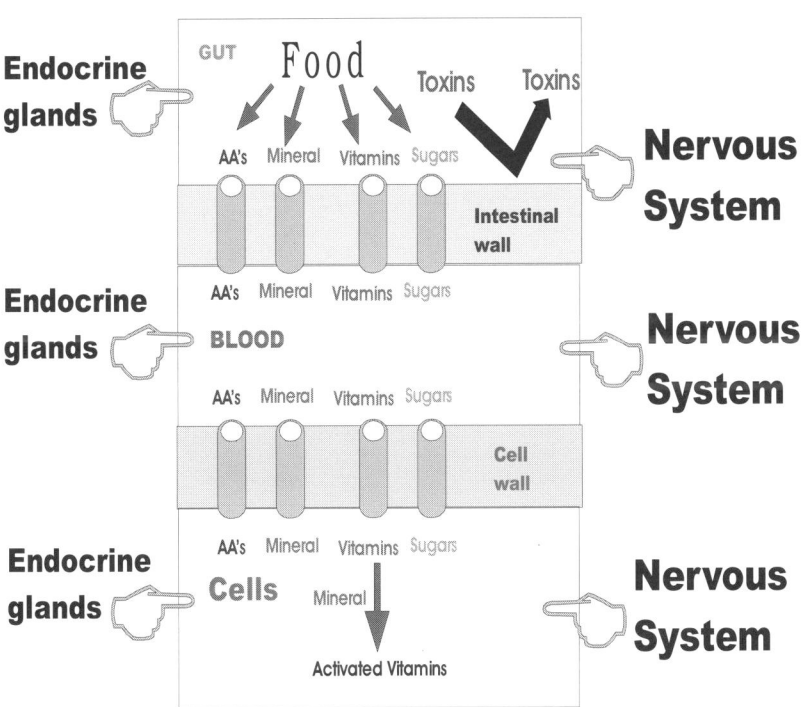

The passage of nutrient flow is determined by the co-operation of the Endocrine and Nervous systems.

Nutrients are "vulnerable" at the activation point

Vitamin

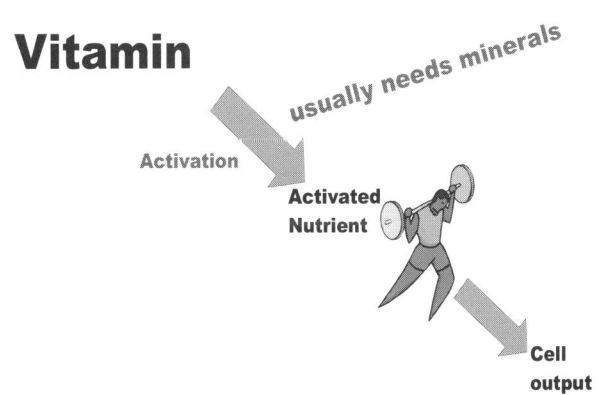

Once Vitamins get into the cells, they need to be activated. Like getting a new credit card. Sign it, ring the 1800 number and only then will it work.

Brain Foods, Brain Poisons

The best-studied examples are the B-Vitamins. It is usually a mineral that is required in the activation stage. Minerals such as Zinc, Magnesium, Molybdenum and Manganese.

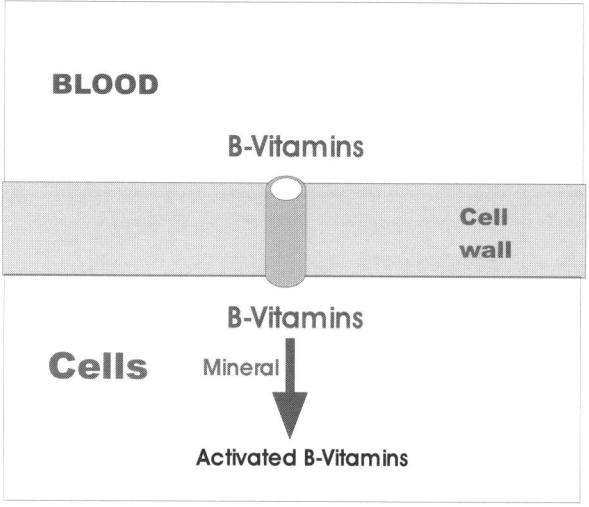

Functional Deficiency Type 1

Functional deficiency Type 1 would involve a Channelopathy and would "starve" the cell of its nutrient. Blood level would be normal or high.

Functional Deficiency Type 2

Functional deficiency Type 2 involves failure to activate the Vitamin due to lack of the activating mineral.

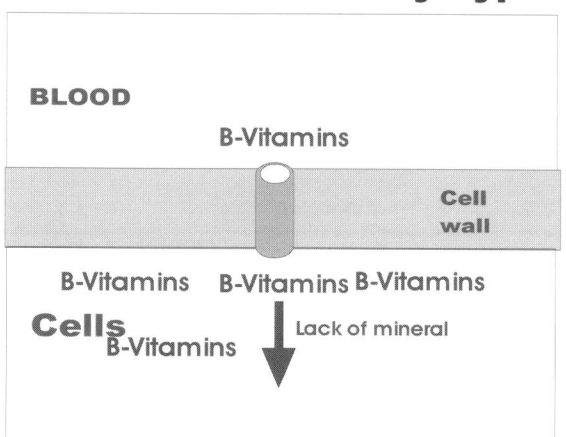

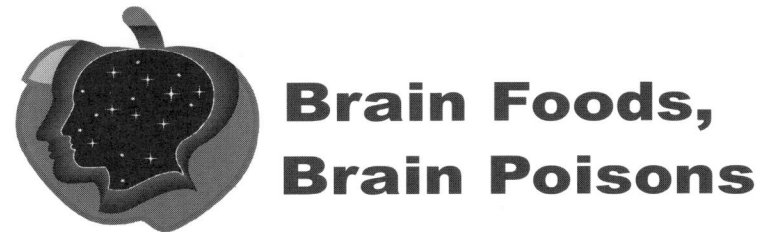 **Brain Foods,
Brain Poisons**

Functional Deficiency Type 3

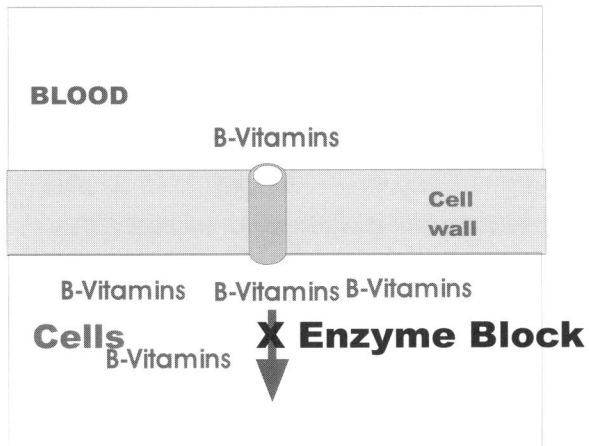

Functional deficiency type 3 would be due to an enzyme block (typically High Copper, Mercury or Lead).

Sites for potential problems with B12- cobalt

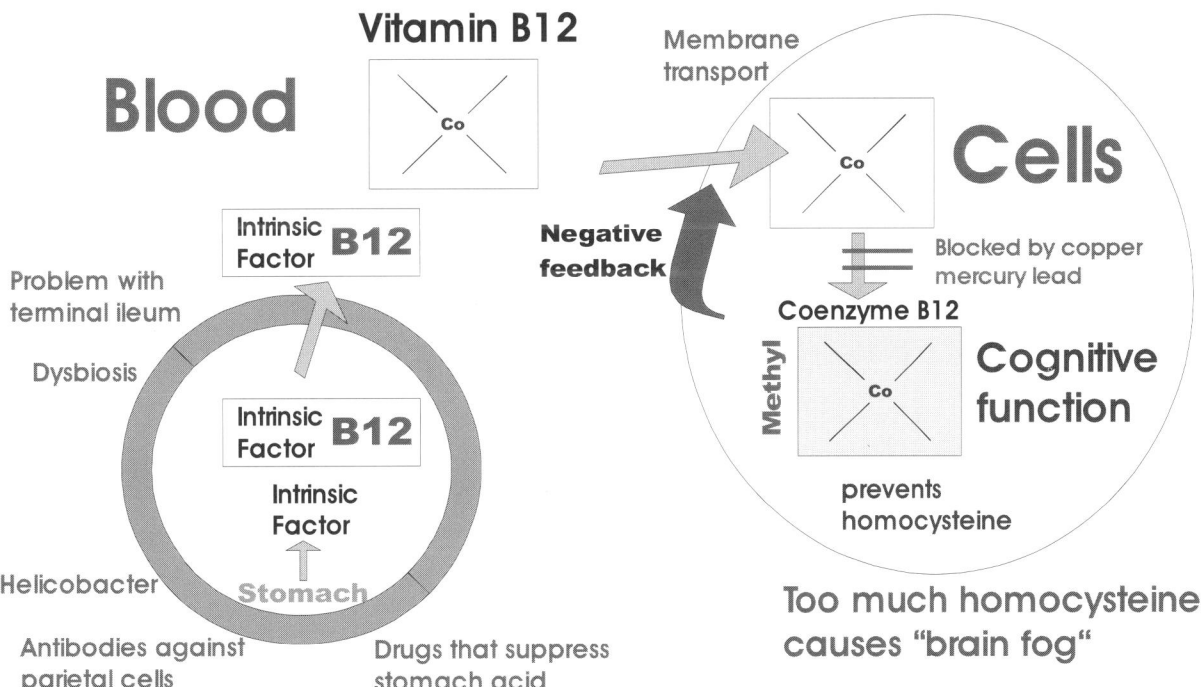

Let's take the example of Vitamin B12. B12 is an unusual marriage of Vitamin and Mineral (cobalt). It enters the blood stream as long as digestive components are present and working properly. Helicobacter and drugs that suppress stomach acid may interfere with this. After reaching the blood it is transported across the cell wall. The "pump" responsible gets turned off when the level of the activated vitamin (Methylcobalamin) is too high. Once in the cell, B12 is "activated" to Methylcobalamin (also called Coenzyme B12). This activated form is responsible for ensuring correct Homocysteine levels in the brain. High brain-cell Homocysteine causes "brain fog", a type of dementia.

Brain Foods, Brain Poisons

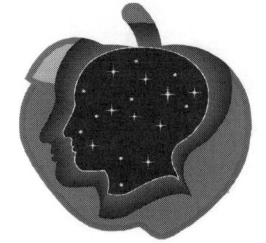

Same biochemistry, different diagnoses

Mercury, Lead or high Copper blocks the conversion, leading to cognitive dysfunction which will get a different label depending on age. Therefore this blockade will lead to normal or high levels of Vitamin B12 in the blood with clear clinical signs of low levels in the tissues. IM injections may prove to be very effective in "getting the brain back" in such patients, especially if the injection is Methylcobalamin.

DSMIV label at different ages

0-2	2-18	18-50	50 plus
Delayed milestones	ADD	Brain fog	Dementia

Functional Deficiency Type 4

Functional Deficiency type 4 involves the late oxidation of the activated vitamin.

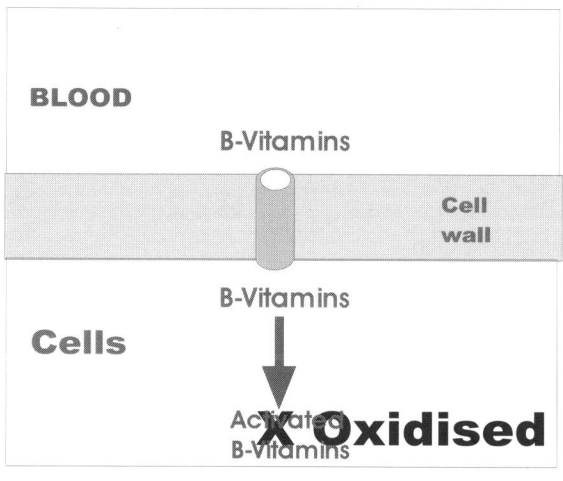

Reasons for divergence

Another way of looking at the abnormalities on TMA is to say that low levels may be caused by Malabsorption (lack of the nutrient) or by Channelopathy (lack of nutrients flowing from the blood to the cells). High levels are due to interference in mineral control systems by toxins.

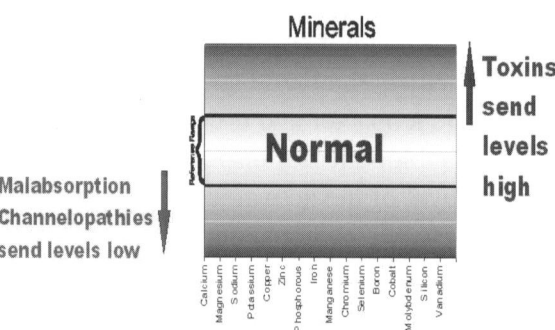

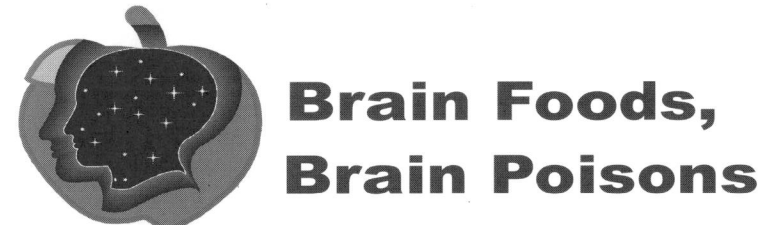

Brain Foods, Brain Poisons

Why toxins may be under-represented

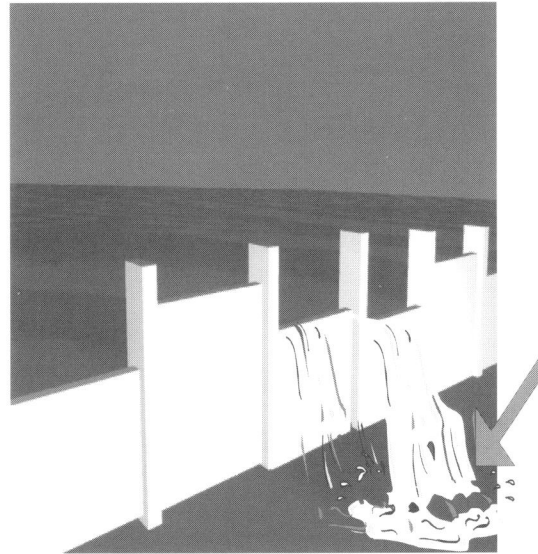

TMA is the "overflow"

The level of toxin on TMA is not proportional to the total body load. Think of the TMA level as the overflow from a dam.

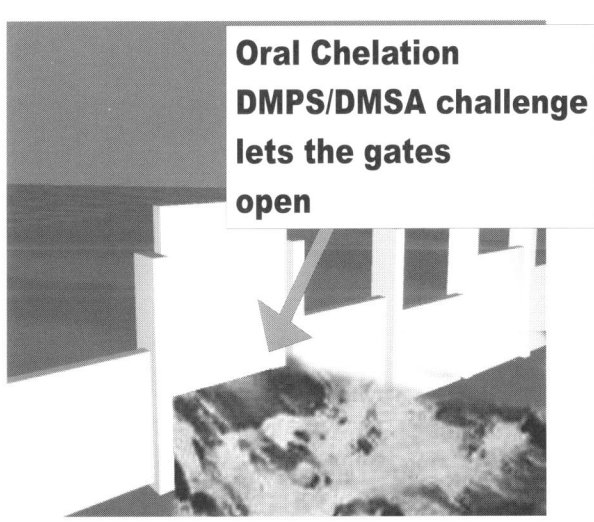

Oral Chelation DMPS/DMSA challenge lets the gates open

Provocation challenges, "let the flood gates open" and subsequent TMA's often show "dormant" toxins coming out.

Each person has a unique journey in time-space

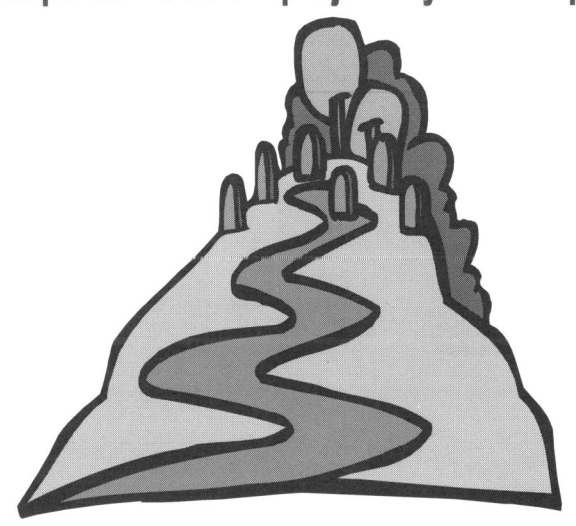

But the question arises, how did the patient get to this point? Each individual has a unique time-space journey (even identical twins).

Brain Foods, Brain Poisons

Time exposure

Two factors are at work here. One is time. At different times in our lives we are exposed to different toxins. Similar to rings of a tree. "In 1947 there was drought, and in 1962 there was a fire".

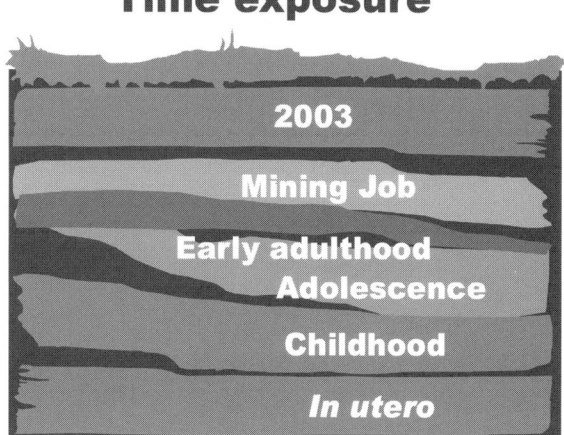

Tissue deposition

These toxins are deposited in different parts of the body depending on genetics, uptake and blood flow.

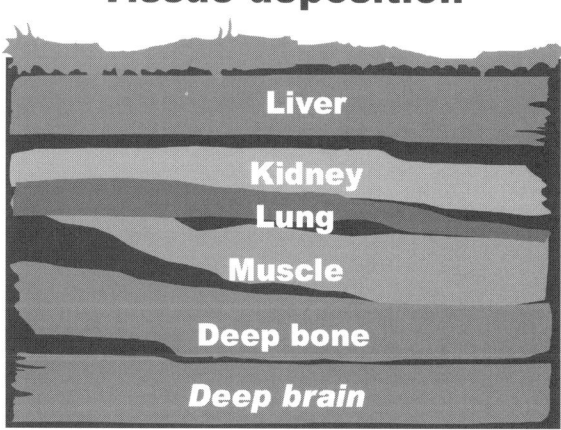

Add the two factors together, and we have an unknown excavation that we are about to embark upon.

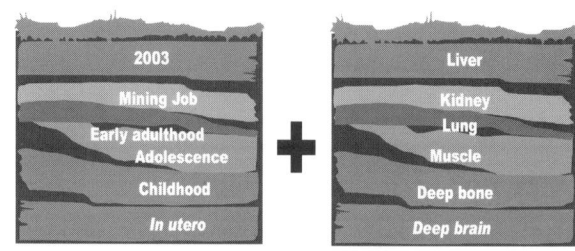

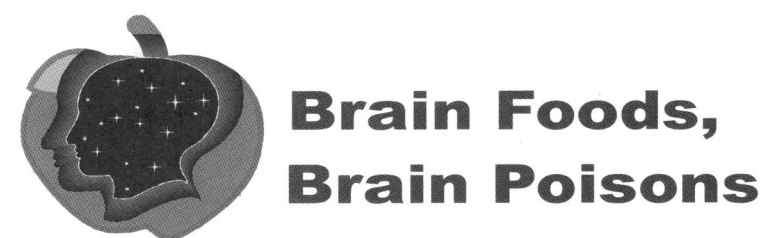

Brain Foods, Brain Poisons

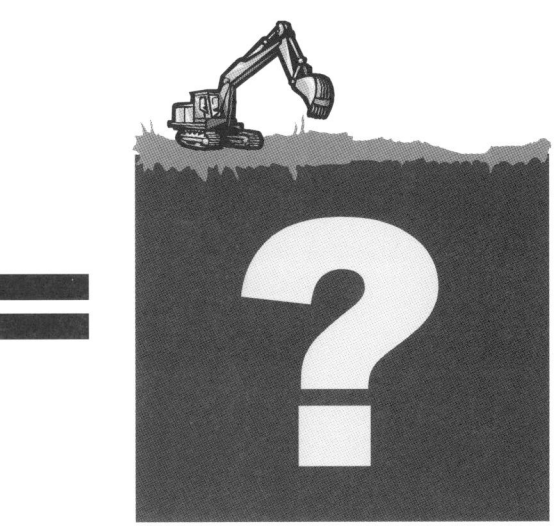

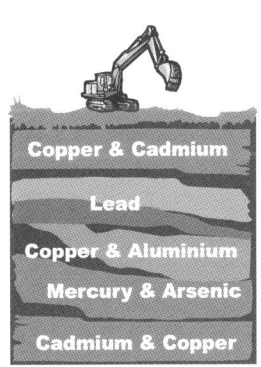

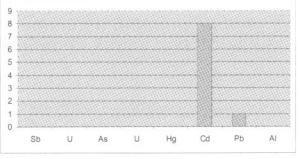

Copper & Cadmium

Lead

Copper & Aluminium

Mercury & Arsenic

Cadmium & Copper

What if the levels looked like this? Then the first TMA "layer" would show only the "surface" toxins coming out, not the full complement.

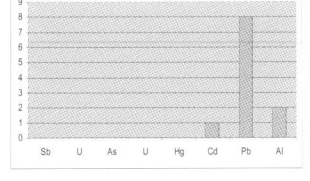

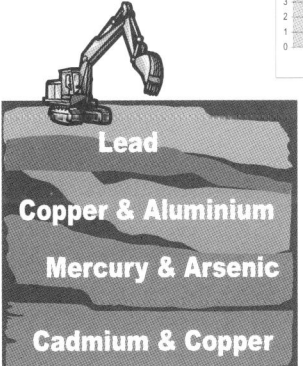

Lead

Copper & Aluminium

Mercury & Arsenic

Cadmium & Copper

The next level would show different toxins.

Brain Foods, Brain Poisons

Each layer has its unique profile of Detox.

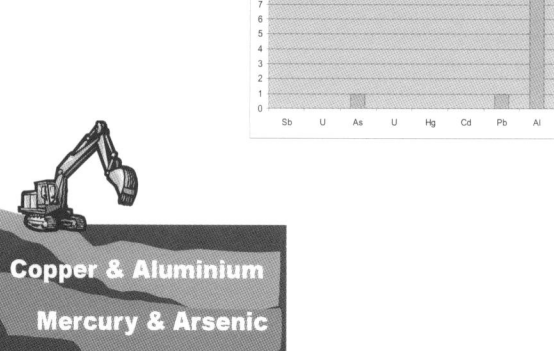

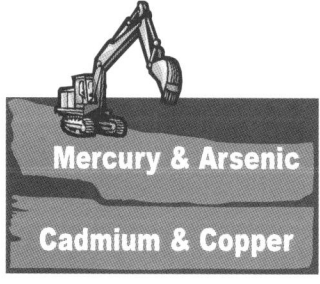

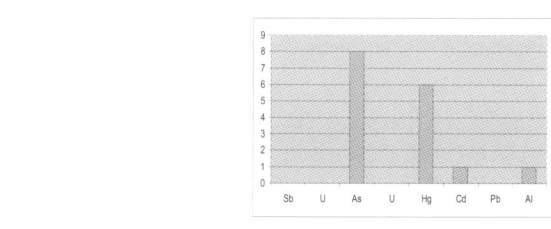

Until we get to the final layer (if that's possible).

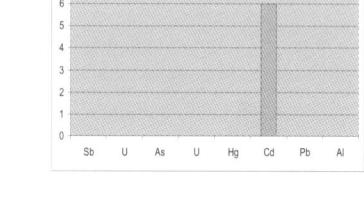

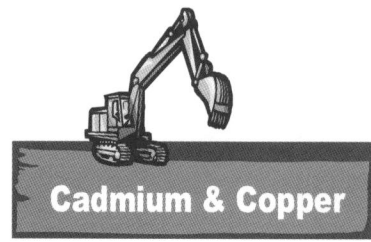

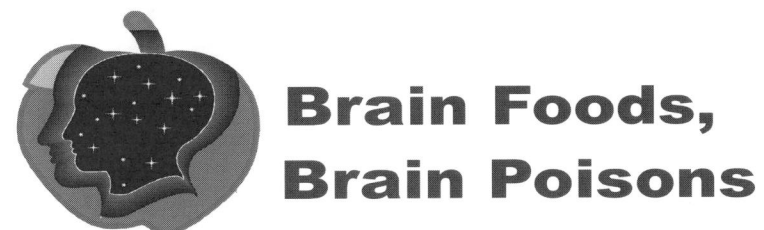

Brain Foods, Brain Poisons

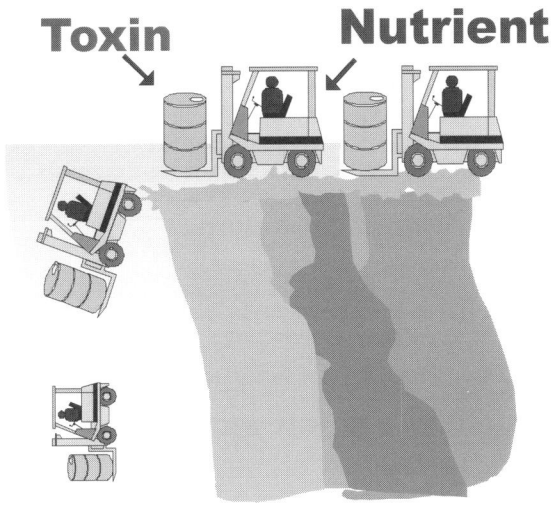

Toxin   **Nutrient**

We also know that nutrients may be "sacrificed" during the Detox process. Extra nutrients will be needed to counteract this effect, to support the body in this journey.

Metabolic observations in Autism

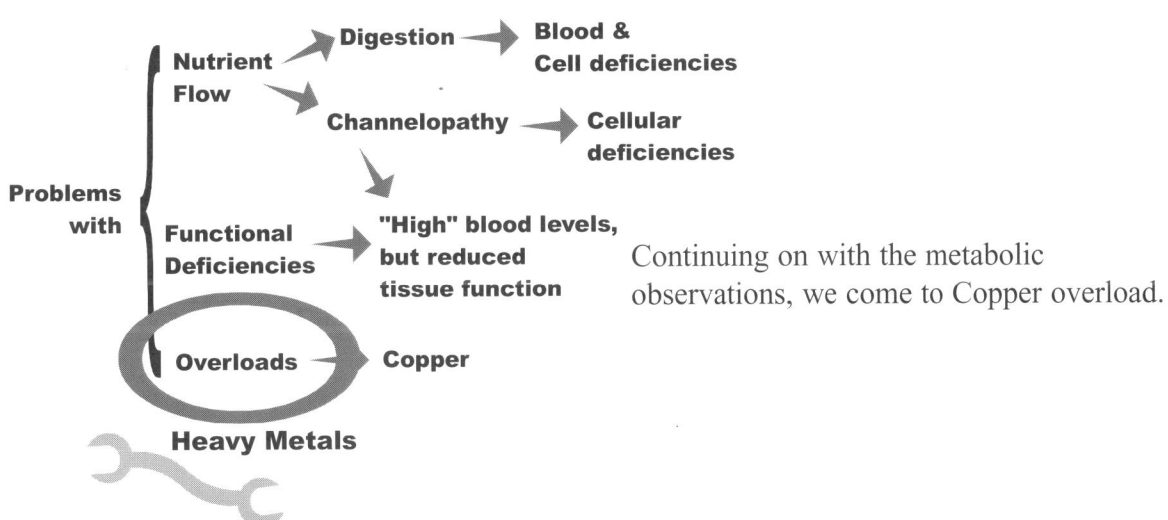

Problems with:
- Nutrient Flow → Digestion → Blood & Cell deficiencies
- → Channelopathy → Cellular deficiencies
- Functional Deficiencies → "High" blood levels, but reduced tissue function
- Overloads → Copper
- Heavy Metals

Continuing on with the metabolic observations, we come to Copper overload.

Organic Toxins in Autism

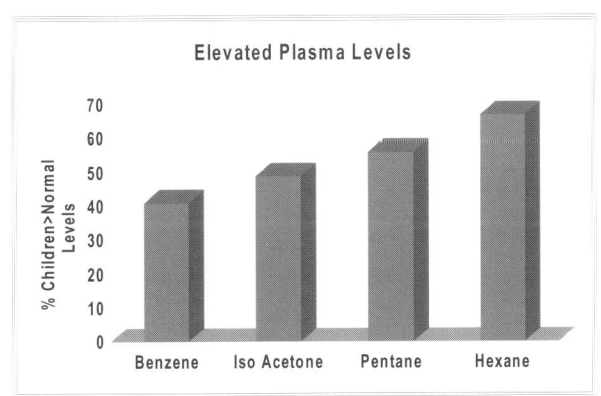

Elevated Plasma Levels

(% Children>Normal Levels: Benzene, Iso Acetone, Pentane, Hexane)

There are many organic toxins found in Autism.

They come under the general classification of

Brain Foods, Brain Poisons

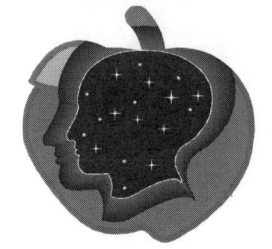

Xenoestrogens

Pesticides	(DDT, DDE, 2,4 5 T, Dieldrin, endosulfan,Dioxins methoxychlor, kepone, toxafene, chloropicrin lindane, chlordane, artrazine)
Metals	Arsenic Cadmium
Petroleum products	(methyl benzine, toluene, car fumes, PCB)
Plastics	(PVC, lunch wraps, etc)
Hormones	a. From Doctors (The Pill & Hormone Replacement therapy) b. From Food 1) Poultry industry 2) Antibiotics in animal feed

Xenoestrogens. "Xeno" meaning stranger. They are "strange" or "false" estrogens, and their prevalence in our lives has increased dramatically in the last 50 years.

So let's talk about Copper. Studies in mammals show that Copper and Iron are stockpiled (particularly in the liver) while the baby is growing. Neonatal Copper is 5-10 times that of an adult. Zinc is the predominant mineral in breast milk to help with growth, immunity and digestion. But Copper and Zinc interact, so Mother Nature decided to stockpile months of Copper and Iron in the baby's liver because to last while Zinc is the main mineral in the diet. It's a very clever system, really.

Prenatal Mineral balance

1] Copper and Iron are "stockpiled" in the liver
   Neonatal liver has 5-10 times
   the adult copper level

2] Zinc is the main mineral in breast milk

   Zinc is for growth
   Zinc is for immunity
   Zinc is for digestion

3] Therefore breast milk is deliberately low
   in Copper & Iron, because they block Zinc

Normal female copper timeline

Balance of Estrogen & Progesterone affects Copper Level

The normal timeline for Copper in women looks a bit like this. Every time Estrogens rise, so does the Copper level. Times like Puberty, taking the Oral Contraceptive Pill, and every pregnancy all change Copper levels. Basically it is the balance of the two hormones Estrogen and Progesterone that determine Copper levels in women.

Puberty	OCP	Pregnancy	Pregnancy	Menopause

Tolerable copper load

Time in years

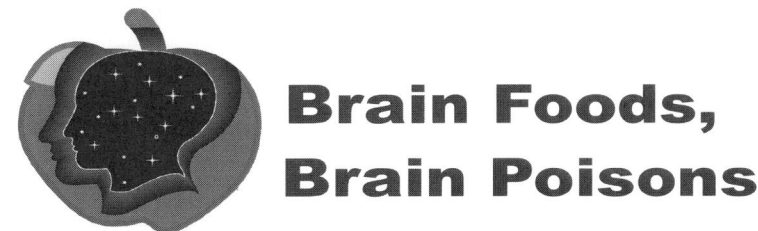

Brain Foods, Brain Poisons

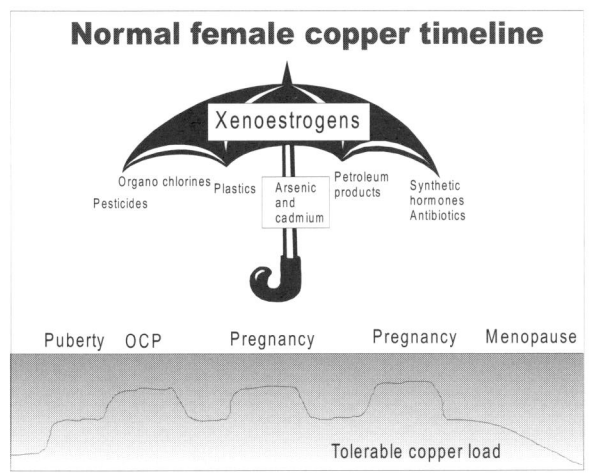

Normal female copper timeline

Xenoestrogens

Organo chlorines Plastics Arsenic and cadmium Petroleum products Synthetic hormones

Pesticides Antibiotics

Puberty OCP Pregnancy Pregnancy Menopause

Tolerable copper load

Time in years

But what if every year we were absorbing more false Estrogens into our bodies?

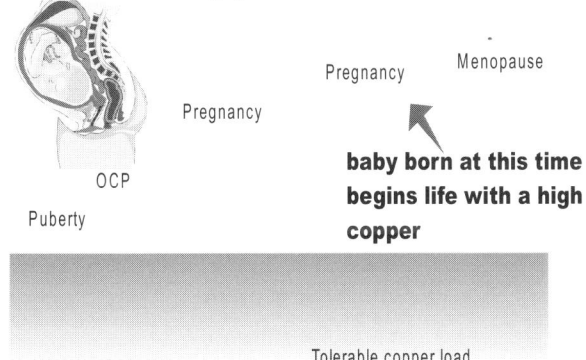

EDS copper timeline

Pregnancy Menopause

Pregnancy

baby born at this time begins life with a high copper

OCP

Puberty

Tolerable copper load

Time in years

The increasing level of these has caused a syndrome called the Estrogen Dominance syndrome (EDS). The article "Why Copper goes up" at the end summaries this.

Each generation, the Copper level is slightly higher, which means that at some point a baby will be born with an intolerable Copper load. Copper is usually disposed of in the bile, but this doesn't happen until the baby is 3 months old!

Zinc & Copper

compete in cells

i.e. High Copper

blocks Zinc in cells

So when we overlay the effect of Copper competition with Zinc, we see that High Copper can produce the same set of symptoms as Zinc deficiency.

Brain Foods, Brain Poisons

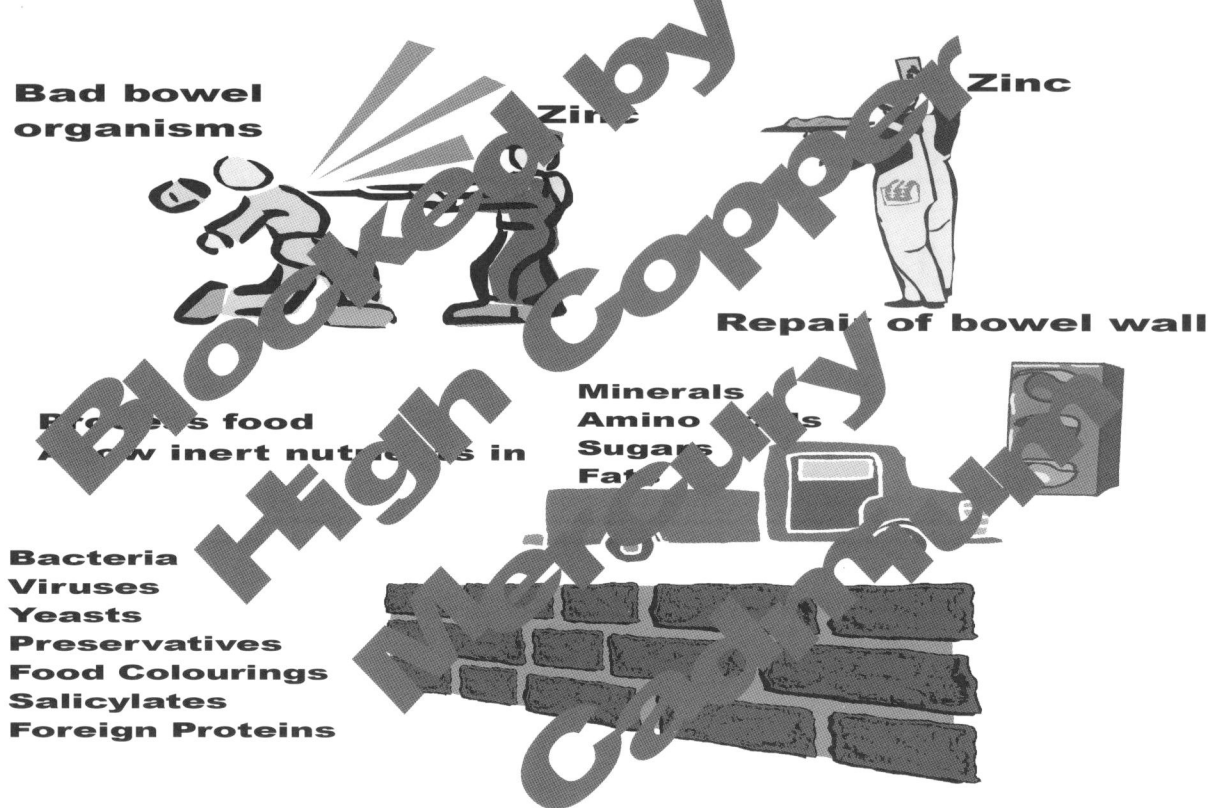

Bad bowel organisms

Zinc

Zinc

Repair of bowel wall

Process food
Allow inert nutrients in

Minerals
Amino acids
Sugars
Fats

Bacteria
Viruses
Yeasts
Preservatives
Food Colourings
Salicylates
Foreign Proteins

This means that many of the digestive symptoms could be due to Copper overload too. Systemic effects of poor digestion are not new ideas in Natural medicine. The clinical consequences of incomplete digestion could fill many a book on naturopathy.

Consequences of poor digestion

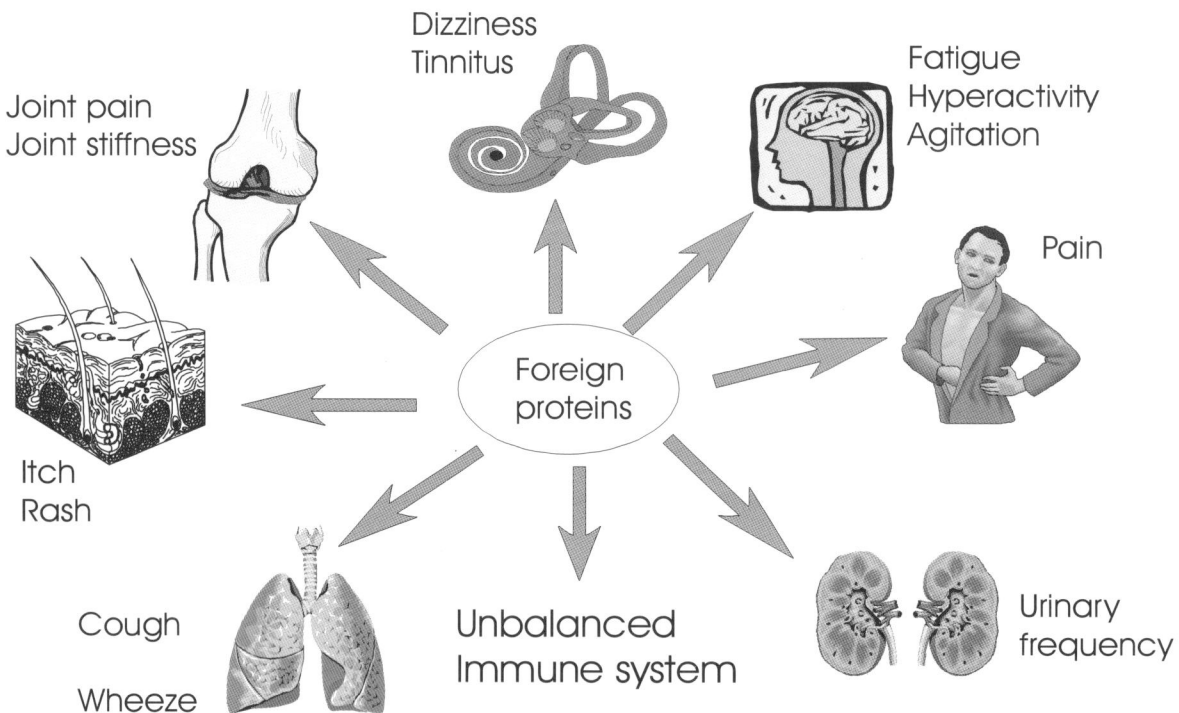

Joint pain
Joint stiffness

Dizziness
Tinnitus

Fatigue
Hyperactivity
Agitation

Pain

Itch
Rash

Foreign proteins

Cough

Wheeze

Unbalanced
Immune system

Urinary
frequency

48

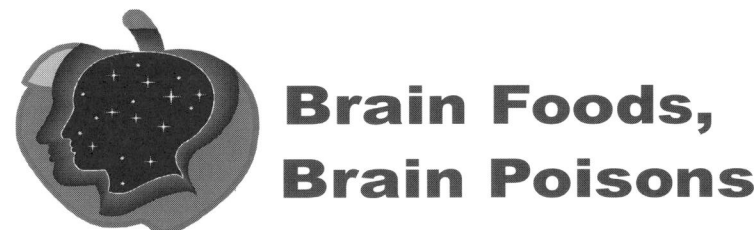

Brain Foods, Brain Poisons

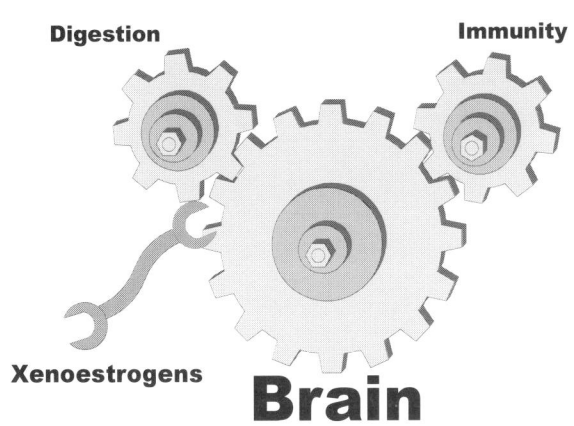

Digestion

Immunity

Xenoestrogens

Brain

So now we have to add the effect of Xenoestrogens (via the increase in Copper) into the digestion equation too.

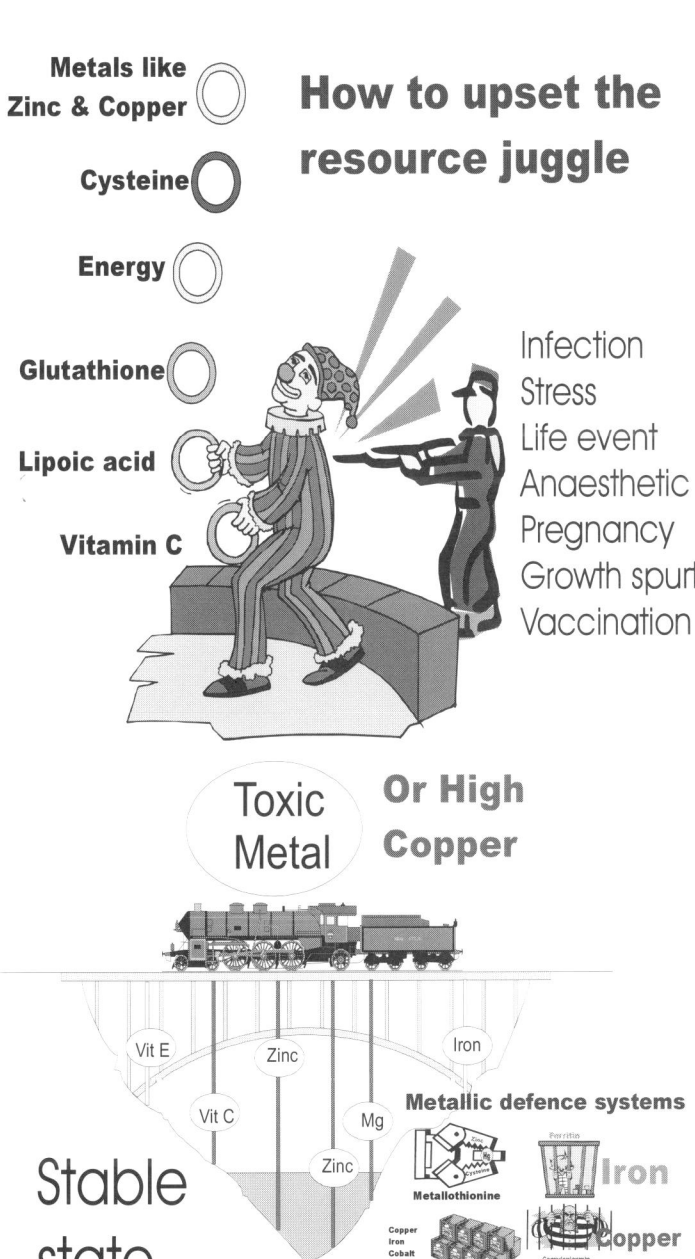

Metals like Zinc & Copper

Cysteine

Energy

Glutathione

Lipoic acid

Vitamin C

How to upset the resource juggle

Infection
Stress
Life event
Anaesthetic
Pregnancy
Growth spurt
Vaccination

The next thing to do would be to consider if vaccination was the only acute insult that could upset the resource juggle. Let's add a few more.

Toxic Metal **Or High Copper**

Stable state

Vit E   Zinc   Iron

Vit C   Mg

Zinc

Metallic defence systems

Metallothionine

Copper
Iron
Cobalt
Manganese
Nickel
Lead   Lipoic acid
Cadmium

Ferritin

Iron

Caeruloplasmin   **Copper**

Glutathione

Let's look at the problem is another way. What if the toxic burden could be likened to the weight of a train on a railway bridge? This is a valid analogy for slowly increasing levels such we see in "Domestic" exposures. As the weight increases, the engineers realise that they cannot rebuild the bridge, so they put up scaffolding in order to support the bridge. Such examples are extra Zinc, Magnesium Iron, Vitamin C, and Vitamin E. Or the metals are contained with our metallic defence system.

Brain Foods, Brain Poisons

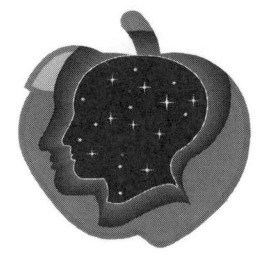

This works well until some acute process uses up the reserves suddenly (the scaffolding gets knocked out). "I'll just borrow this for a few minutes, and bring it right back!" Sound familiar?

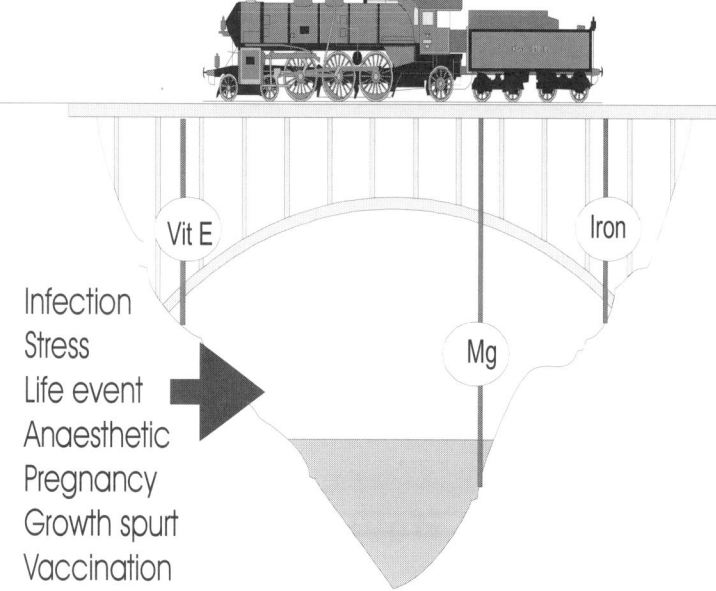

Vit E

Iron

Mg

Infection
Stress
Life event
Anaesthetic
Pregnancy
Growth spurt
Vaccination

Collapsed state

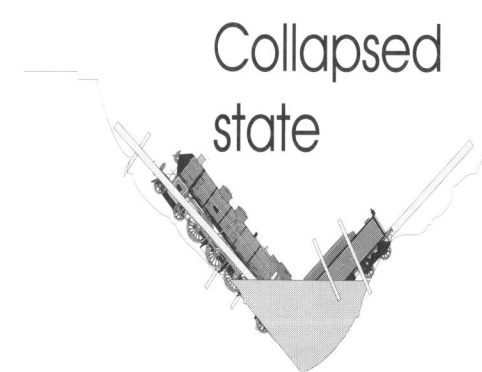

Then the system collapses. It is at this point the symptoms occur.

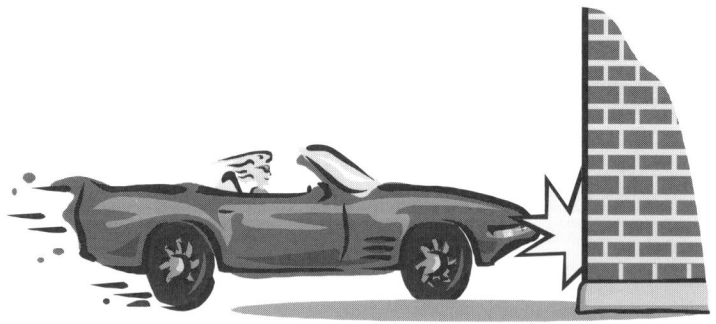

Or to put it another way when we crashed, the air bag has not gone off.

Antioxidant air-bag

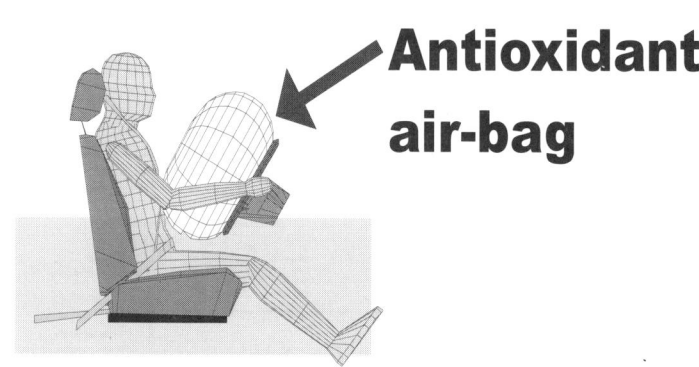

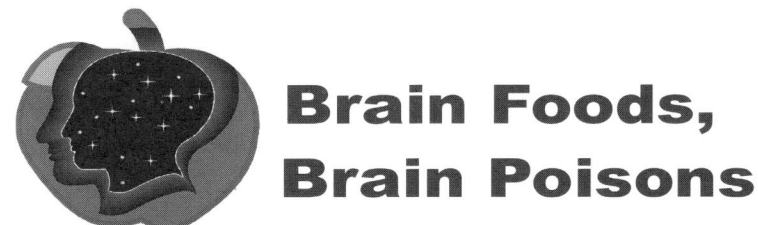

Brain Foods, Brain Poisons

Metabolic observations in Autism

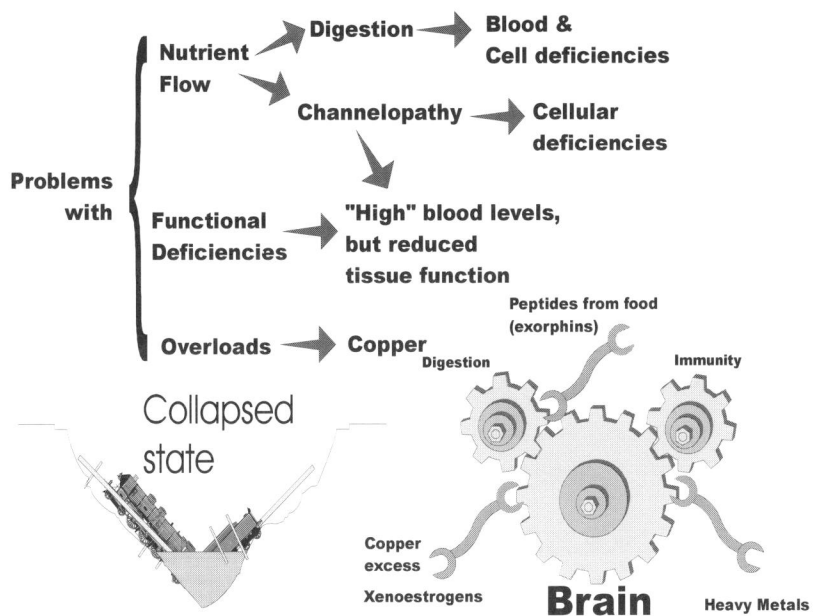

Now put all the observations together. A pre-existing vulnerable state has preceded the acute insult. A pre-existing state like a compensated toxic or overloaded system. The collapsed state unmasks the oxidative stress, but it can't correct itself quickly enough due to lack of resources or ineffective resources.

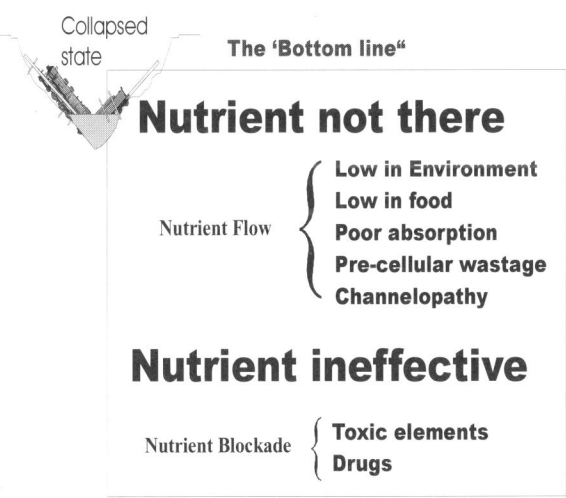

In the collapsed state we determine the "bottom line".

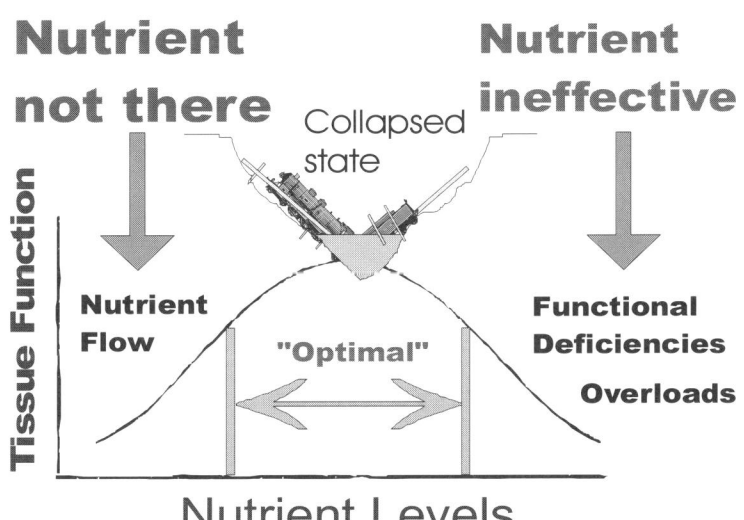

We overlay the symptoms by analysis of the nutrients out of range.

Brain Foods, Brain Poisons

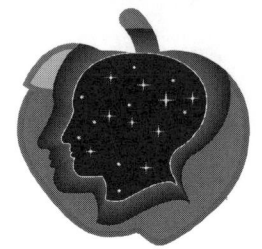

DOM investigative approach

What is the process that caused this?

Tissue Function (vertical axis)

Process ?

X X X X

Nutrient Levels

Autism Spectrum Disorder

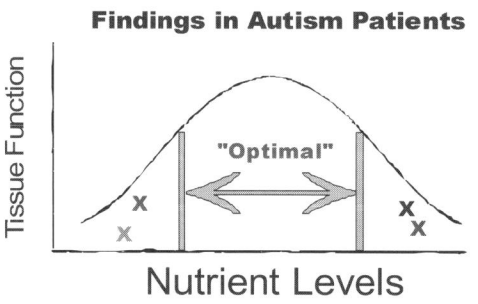

Collapsed state

The four observations can now be analysed as a process, not just as metabolic changes.

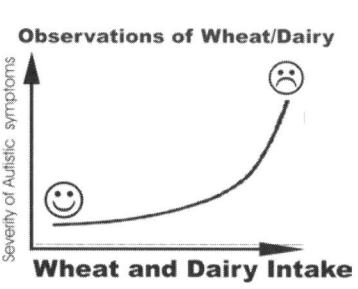

Peptides from food (exorphins)

Digestion

Immunity

Copper excess Xenoestrogens

Brain

Heavy Metals

Findings in Autism Patients

Tissue Function (vertical axis)

"Optimal"

X X X X

Nutrient Levels

Observations of Wheat/Dairy

Severity of Autistic symptoms (vertical axis)

Wheat and Dairy Intake

WHY?

Buy why has it happened?

1] Escalating levels of environmental toxins

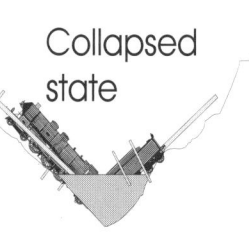

Collapsed state

2] Prenatal maternal toxins

3] Post-natal oxidative stress

4] Final destabilising insult

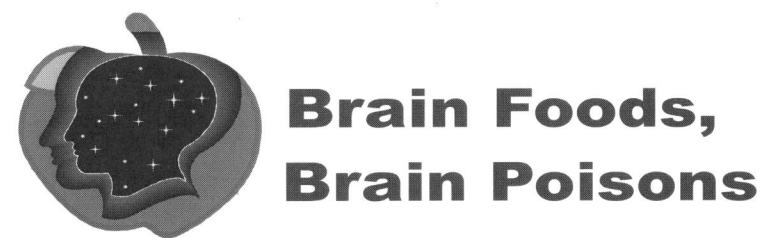

Detoxification Observations

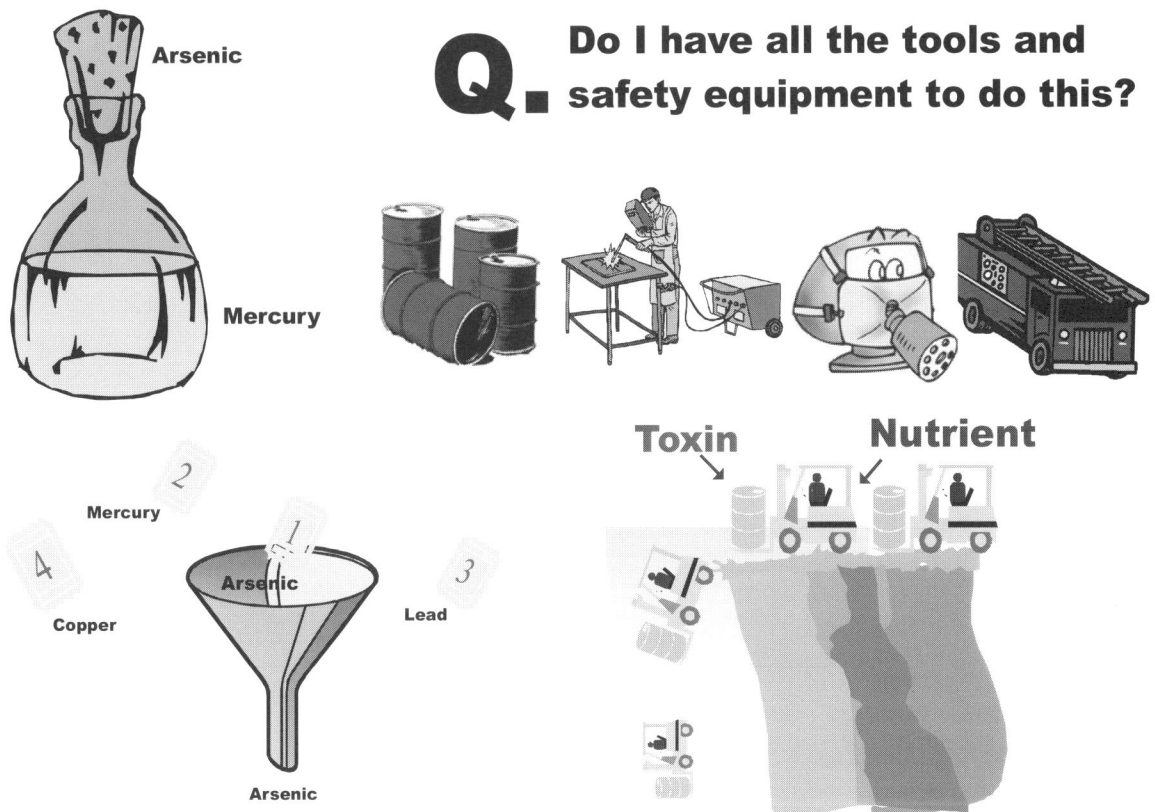

Q. Do I have all the tools and safety equipment to do this?

Arsenic

Mercury

Mercury

Copper

Arsenic

Lead

Arsenic

Toxin

Nutrient

Autism protocols frequently contain detox treatments. As we set about to detoxify, what factors could determine the reaction to such procedures and the time-course of such procedures?

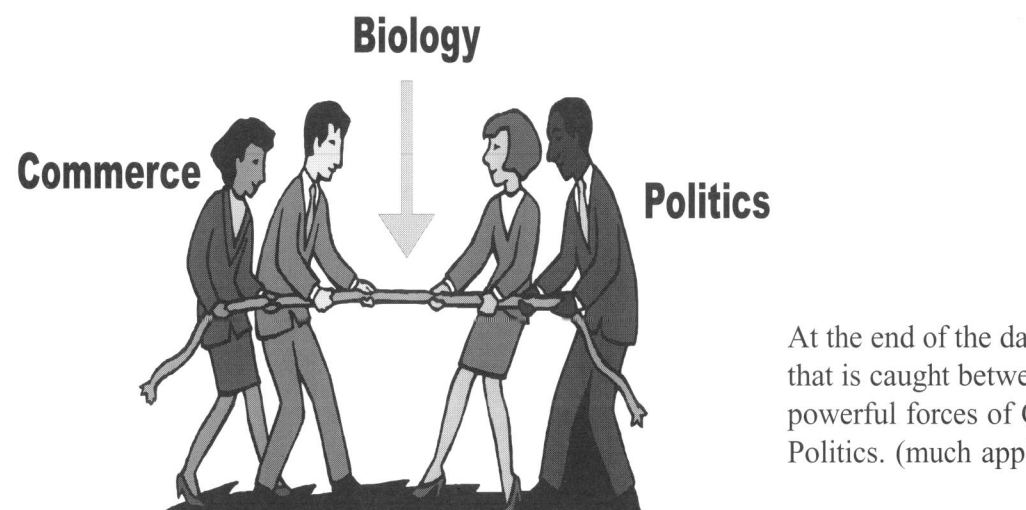

Biology

Commerce

Politics

At the end of the day it is biology that is caught between the two powerful forces of Commerce and Politics. (much applause).

An important aspect of Nutritional Medicine relates to the metallic containment systems that have evolved especially relating to charged ions. Bulk ions get lots of airplay in medical schools, but infact play *very little* part in enzyme functions. Microminerals however carry out most of the enzymatic reactions, but get extremely little mention in medical school curricula. Perhaps their teachers stopped reading after 1960?

Charged ions

"Bulk" ions low Mol Wt

Sodium
Potassium
Calcium

Strong
containment
systems

VERY few
enzymes
use these
as cofactors !!!!!!

Microminerals

Magnesium
Zinc
Iron
Copper
Manganese
Molybdenum
Selenium
Chromium
Cobalt

Mostly cations (two plus charge)
Electron donors
Containment systems <u>except</u> Mg

Hundreds
of enzymes
use these
as cofactors!!!!!!

The importance of these containment systems was aptly summarized by Professor Bilinski. What we need then is *some* of these minerals, but not *too many* of them in the wrong place. Despite what vitamin supplement companies push, it is clear that more is *not* better!

In order to deal with them (divalent cations) we have a system that can store them and release them

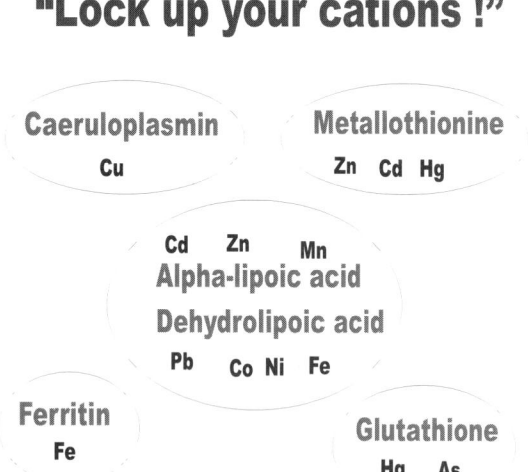

"Lock up your cations !"

Caeruloplasmin
Cu

Metallothionine
Zn Cd Hg

Cd Zn Mn
Alpha-lipoic acid
Dehydrolipoic acid
Pb Co Ni Fe

Ferritin
Fe

Glutathione
Hg As

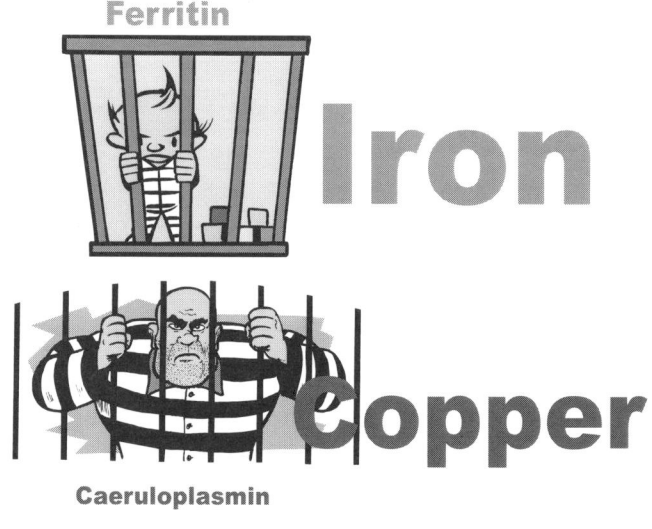

Ferritin

Iron

Caeruloplasmin

Copper

Metallothionine Structure

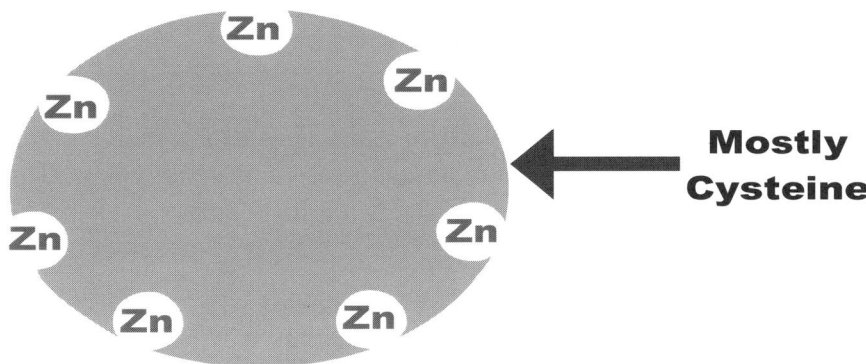

Better-known examples are ferritin and caeruloplasmin for containing copper and iron. Copper and iron have high electro negativities and pose real problems to cells that wish to use them safely.

Another metalloprotein is Metallothionine, which is predominantly the sulfurous amino acid cysteine with seven zinc atoms. This compound forms part of defence system against heavy metals and too much copper. It is distributed in the gastrointestinal tract, skin, liver and brain. Disorders of it cause symptoms ranging from dairy intolerance to autism. See the chapter on zinc for more on this.

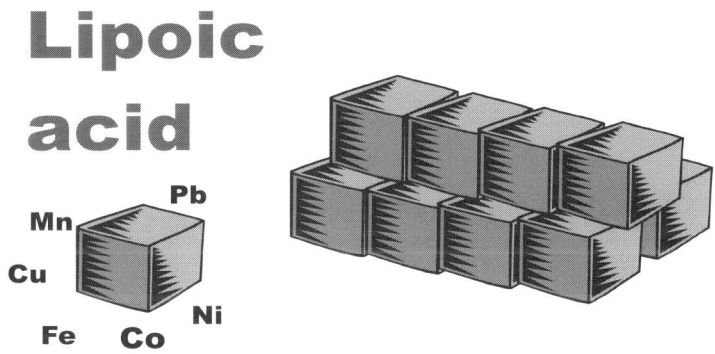

Another containment system is Alpha Lipoic Acid (ALA). ALA can complex with most divalent cations (2 plus positive ionic charge atoms). It is a valuable method of metal control within cells.

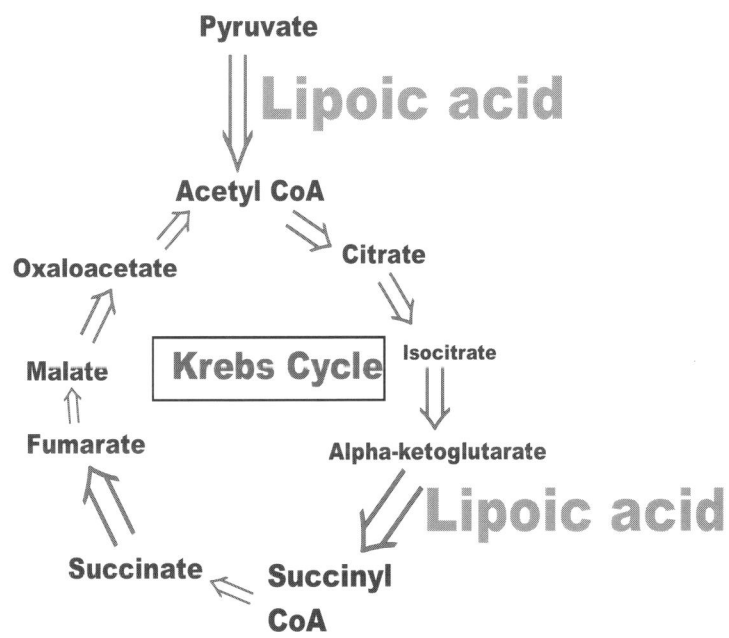

That is, if you can *spare* some of it from the Krebs cycle. This means that there may be a resource management problem for cells facing both oxidative stress and toxic metals. This could lead to neuro-degenerative conditions like Alzheimer's and Multiple Sclerosis.

Cells utilize nutrients in 3 ways; Storage/ Structure, Enzyme functions and charge/pH management. Activated nutrients utilization often defines the output of the cell. It is integral to what it does.

There are various mechanisms of intracellular antagonism and the offending atoms are listed with the nutrients they block or destroy on page 14. This is why one must know the level of *both* molecules in order to know how symptoms are being generated. The most potent blockade is by Mercury, then Cadmium.

As toxins arrive, they are stored in various parts of the cell, often inadvertently with a nutrient. This may "tie up" nutrients which get involved with this misuse. It may mean that higher levels are needed to function because normal levels "cancel out" in the presence of toxins. The analogy is like needing to use more accelerator if you have the parking brake stuck on. Antagonism of Zinc by mercury is said to be 1000:1 and Cadmium 100:1.

Cellular defence system

Blood

Aluminium   Mercury   Cadmium   Antimony   Lead

Aluminium   Mercury   Cadmium   Antimony   Antimony

Tissues

Zinc Zinc Zinc
Mercury Zinc
Cadmium Zinc
Antimony Zinc
Aluminium Zinc

Chromium
Chromium Chromium
Chromium
Lead Chromium

Iron Iron
Iron
Iron **Lead**
Iron
Iron **Mercury**
Iron

56

A theme which readers may have picked up from my articles relates to the concept of balance within biological systems. This is a feature of eastern medicine, which is generally not incorporated into western science, perhaps with the exception of physics. Balance can be described as "when two opposing components create equilibrium in a biological system". In other words, these can be naturally opposing components like zinc and copper or a nutrient and its counteracting *antinutrient* such as zinc and cadmium. A list below shows examples of such nutrient antinutrient combinations.

Anti-nutrients

Lead blocks Iron Calcium Molybdenum Manganese Chromium Sulphur Cobalt

Mercury blocks Zinc selenium iron sulphur cobalt transmembrane ion channels

Cadmium blocks Zinc Magnesium Selenium Sulphur

Arsenic blocks Vit E selenium sulphur boron

Aluminium blocks Vit E Vit C Vit B1 Zinc Selenium Sodium Potassium Phosphorus

Antimony blocks Zinc Selenium

In this situation, minerals are somewhat easier to understand because we could mentally imagine one mineral blocking anothers function within an enzyme. What is poorly understood is that Antinutrients can cause havoc within cells without being labelled as toxic i.e. below "toxic" levels. The definitions of toxicity are primarily defined by industry, not medicine. These industries wish to define toxicity by the least sensitive method of detection. Tissue mineral analysis is the most sensitive method of detection of heavy metals; hence industry will not use this tool. This spills over into the medical profession, who cannot understand why hair analysis is so useful for the improvement of health.

Very important Concept

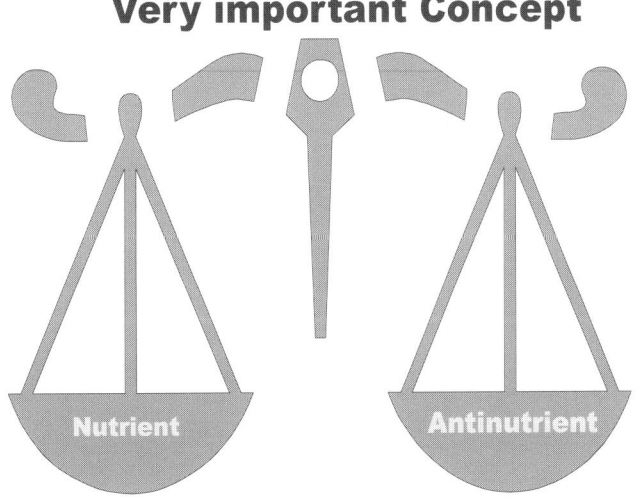

The point is this: you cannot understand the level of a nutrient unless you measure its *opposing* component. For instance, a normal ferritin in the presence of lead, will still give symptoms of iron deficiency. A normal red cell zinc in the presence of excess copper will still give the symptoms of zinc deficiency. A normal red cell magnesium in the presence of cadmium will still give symptoms of magnesium deficiency. Just measuring the blood levels and making assumptions about the opposing component *will not always work*. In fact it may lead to unnecessary and prolonged supplementation, with the eventual increasing of dose to control symptoms. If the copper is rising, then you need more Vitamin C over time to prevent say bleeding gums.

Balance is not just a simple set of scales; it involves three or four-dimensions. The figure below shows that copper, zinc, magnesium and molybdenum need to be in balance for correct energy cycles. Abnormalities of this tetrahedron and the main problem in chronic fatigue syndrome. Another figure shows the balance between magnesium, sodium, potassium and calcium. The balance of this tetrahedron determines nervous system function. When one combines the two, with magnesium in the centre, we see that alterations in one eventually lead to a change in the other tetrahedral balance. *These balances cannot be determined by blood test*. Only a tissue sample will provide this type of

Mineral balance and function

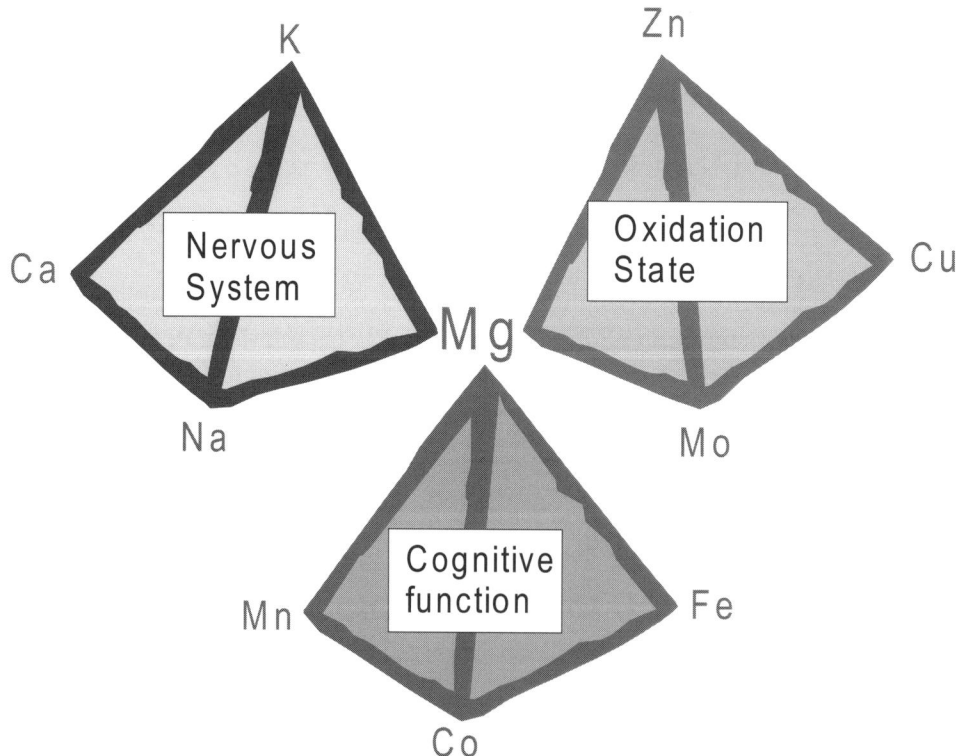

information. Biochemistry occurs in the tissues, not the blood. More importantly the solution requires understanding *why* the imbalance occurred and at which point, did disruption occur.

Nutrients and antinutrients

	Copper block	Cadmium Block	Mercury Block	Arsenic Block	Lead Block	Aluminium Block	Antimony Block
Sodium						X	
Potassium						X	
Magnesium	X	X					
Calcium					X		
Iron	X		X		X		
Zinc	X	X	X			X	X
Chromium					X		
Selenium		X	X	X		X	X
Molybdenum	X				X		
Manganese	X						
Phosphorus						X	
Vitamin B1	X					X	
Vitamin C	X					X	
Vitamin E	X			X		X	
Folate	X						

The roles of Hair analysis and health questionnaires.

The questionnaire gives the practitioner an historical profile of symptoms. By examining these with the hair analysis (TMA), we can gauge what minerals are low or being disrupted. In addition to a blood test they reveal a process underlying the progression of the illness.

Ordinarily our bodies work transparently to us, just like using a motorcar. We turn the key, the engine starts and we never have to understand about transistors, ignition, fuel injection, pistons, exhausts etc. We only take note when something goes wrong. Bodies are the same. Symptoms are cells crying out for help. Just like babies, if we can decode the cry, we can deduce why the baby is crying. There are 4 reasons why they might cry.

1] Reduced intake. 2] Rapid loss 3] Poor tissue uptake. 4] Intracellular blockade. The key to analysing a nutritional problem is to find out what is the process that has affected nutrient flow.

The 'Bottom line"

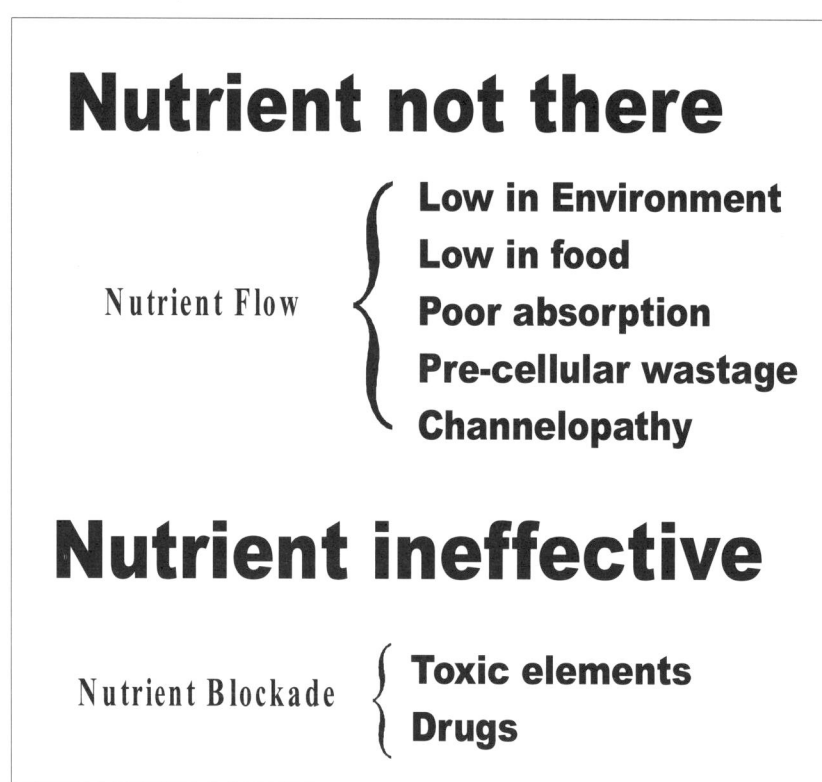

Nutrient not there

Nutrient Flow
{
Low in Environment
Low in food
Poor absorption
Pre-cellular wastage
Channelopathy

Nutrient ineffective

Nutrient Blockade
{
Toxic elements
Drugs

The bottom line is that there are 2 ways to generate symptoms. Either the nutrient isn't there or it is blocked by something. Traditional approaches that concentrate on deficiencies are totally out of date. They ignore the vast work of Tissue mineral science and metallotoxicology.

You cannot understand the level of a nutrient unless you measure its *opposing* component. For instance, a normal ferritin in the presence of lead, will still give symptoms of iron deficiency. A normal red cell zinc in the presence of excess copper will still give the symptoms of zinc deficiency. A normal red cell magnesium in the presence of cadmium will still give symptoms of magnesium deficiency. Just measuring the blood levels and making assumptions about the opposing component *will not always work*. In fact it may lead to unnecessary and prolonged supplementation, with the eventual increasing of dose to control symptoms. If the copper is rising, then you need more Vitamin C over time to prevent say bleeding gums.

The rules of reading a TMA are listed below

Rules of Hair analysis

Low is deficient
(in some tissues)
High is a message
Copper is common
Toxins maybe hidden
(until next sample)

Actually all variations from the reference range are messages. These messages point to processes that fall outside the diagnostic capabilities of most doctors. This is why high levels are messages rather than a true reflection of tissue storage.

Reasons for divergence

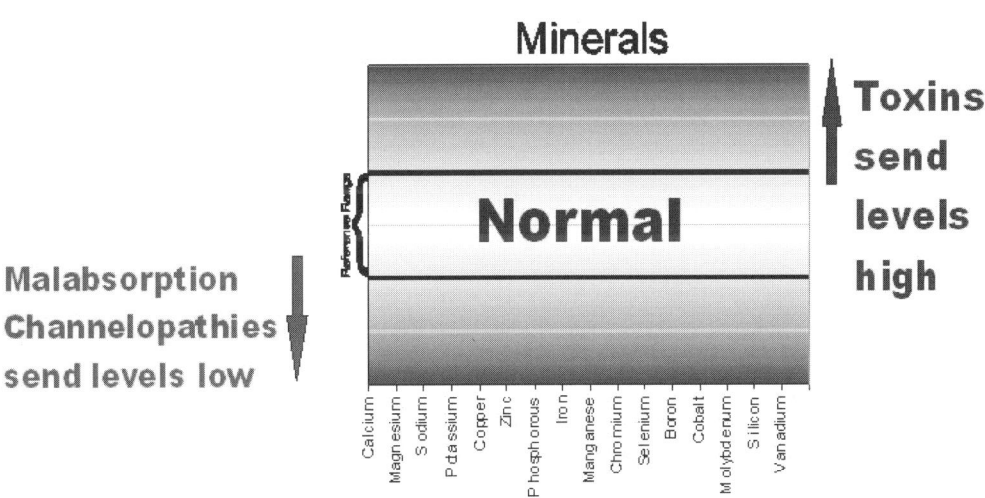

	Effect	
Toxin	**TMA**	**Symptoms**
Aluminium	Na, K, P	Zinc, Vitamin C
Antimony		Zinc Selenium
Arsenic	Boron	Vitamin E
Cadmium	Zinc, Mg Ca	Zinc Magnesium
Copper excess	Mg, Mn, Boron	Zinc Mg Vitamin C
Lead	Ca, Fe, Mo, Cr, Na, K	Iron
Mercury	Cobalt, low K	Zinc Iron

Need both to solve clinical puzzles

Minerals

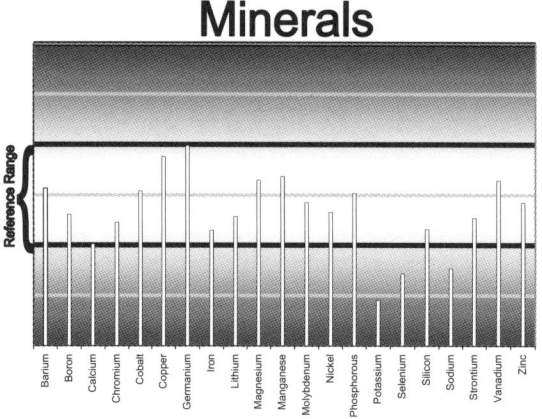

Reference Range

Barium | Boron | Calcium | Chromium | Cobalt | Copper | Germanium | Iron | Lithium | Magnesium | Manganese | Molybdenum | Nickel | Phosphorous | Potassium | Selenium | Silicon | Sodium | Strontium | Vanadium | Zinc

Hair sample

Disruption to minerals

Health Questionnaire Please complete all 3 pages

Name: .... D.O.B. ....

Address..

NRS

What is the *main reason* for attending our clinic?........................

Please tick the appropriate column

Topic	Have you had......	never	In the past	Recently	frequently
Digestion	Heartburn or reflux				
	Bloating after meals				
	Constipation				
	Burping, Farting or wind				
	diarrhoea or loose stools				
	Nausea (feeling like vomiting)				
	Stomach ulcers or Stomach pain				
	Gall bladder problems				
Lung	Asthma or Emphysema				
	Pneumonia or Bronchitis				
	Wheeze after viral infection				
	Wheeze after exercise				
Immune system	Boils or pimples				
	Cold sores				
	Conjunctivitis				
	Ear infection				
	Genital infection				
	Mouth ulcers				
	Sinus infection				
	Sore throat				
	Thrush				
	Tonsillitis				
	Urinary infection				
Skin, Hair & Nails	Acne or pimples				
	Brittle nails				
	Dry eyes or mouth				
	Dry skin				
	Eczema or Dermatitis				
	Early greying of hair				
	Hair loss				
	Psoriasis				
	Rashes				
	Sore or cracked lips				
	Tinea or ringworm				
	Stretch marks				
	White spots on nails				
	Warts				

Do you have allergies?

Allergy		No	Yes		
	Medications			list ....
	Foods or herbs			list ....
	Hay fever or sinus trouble			
	Nasal blockage			
	Other			list ....

Gynaecological		never	In the past	Recently	frequently
	Abnormal PAP smears				
	Breast Cyst or lumps				
	Breast tenderness				
	Endometriosis				
	Fibroids				
	Ovarian cysts				
	PMS/PMT				
	been on HRT				
	been on oral contraceptive				

Questionnaire

Symptom clusters

Some interesting research from the chronic fatigue syndrome literature has revealed a set of conditions called Channelopathies. The name refers to the ion channels that allow metallic ions in and out of the cell, but could be applied more broadly to the passage of Nutrients into the cell and the release of Toxins out of the cell. The best-known example of Channelopathy is Cystic Fibrosis due to an abnormality of chromosome 7. This involves the "chloride" channel.

Some specific examples would include well-known one-way channels such as inflowing potassium

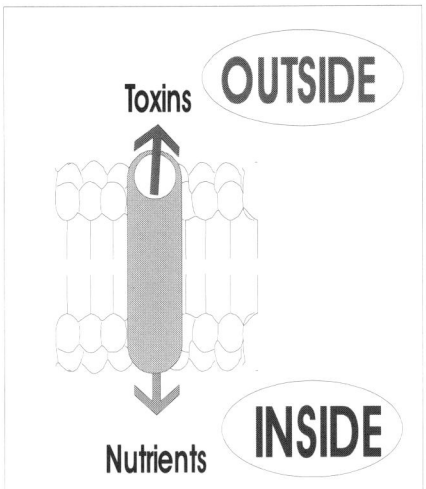

and the anti-port (counter pump) system of Sodium and Potassium. Of note is that Magnesium is required for one of these Potassium channels and Vitamin B6 is needed for the Na/K Anti-port pump.

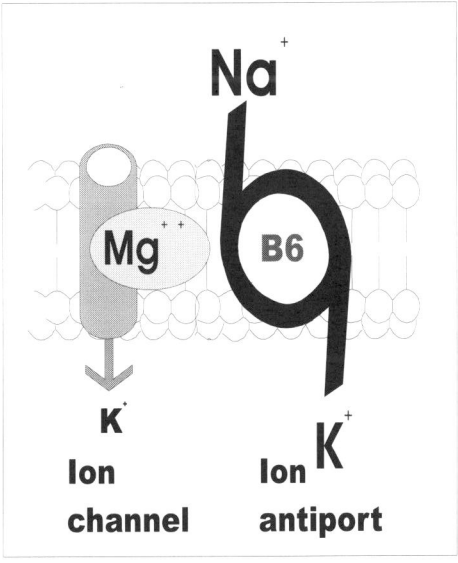

If we take a look at the passage from the gut to the cells, we see 2 important hurdles that need to be traversed. The Intestinal wall, and the target cell wall and in the case of the brain, the glial cells.

It is well known that glutamine is helpful for the intestinal wall passage while taurine is useful for the target cell wall passage. In general Amino Acids may play important roles in ion "delivery" systems, and this explains why some patients do better on Amino Acid Chelate supplements.

A common channelopathy is the disruption to the Na/K pump due to organophosphate pesticides. Organochlorines probably affect Cu/K or Cu/Mo pumps. This explains why such pesticides cause copper retention disorders.

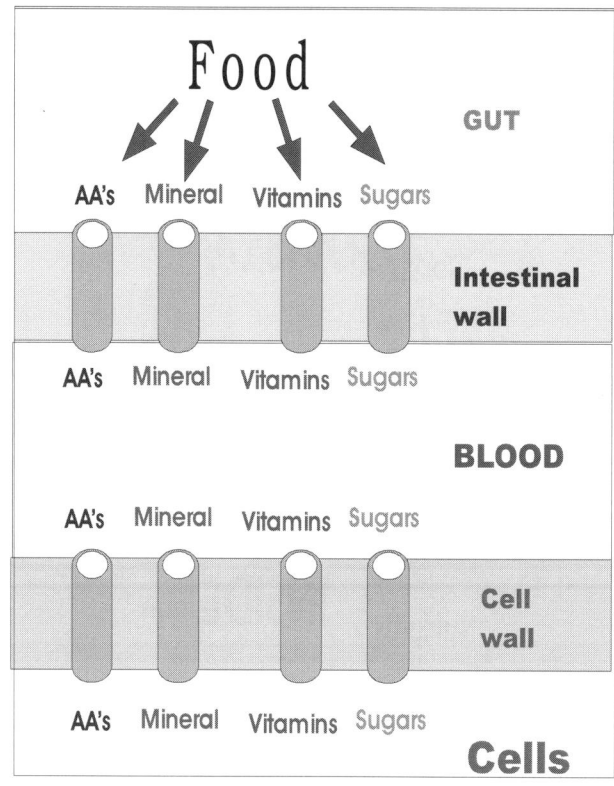

Interestingly, these channels sit in "vats" of oil including the essential fatty acids (EFA's). The oils vary with blood group. When we test a person's blood group we subject the surface of the cell to a biochemical reaction and depending on the reaction we determine the blood group. This means that the cell wall is different for each blood group and this difference is actually coded for on Chromosome 9. The table below summarises the different Omega 3, 6 & 9 requirements according to blood group. AB group's need the same as B, which are Flax seed oil capsules. These oils have been used in many conditions and may be diagnosistic in some Channelopathies at 6 to 9 grams per day.

Essential Fatty Acids (EFA's)

Blood Group			
	A	Ω 3	Fish oil
	O	Ω 3 & 6	Evening Primrose oil Borage or Starflower
	B	Ω 3, 6 & 9	Flaxseed oil

Channelopathy is a problem with channels

Why Copper goes up.

Most of my patients when confronted with their high coppers usually react by saying "impossible"; I've never ingested copper in my life. The list below shows a comprehensive group of foods that contain copper. Bee Pollen, Buckwheat, Oats, Wheat Bran, Wheat Germ, Butter, Eggs, Apples, Apricot Kernels, Bananas, Olives, Oranges, Peaches, Prunes, Raisins, Mushrooms Burdock, Chickweed, Cocoa, Dandelion Greens, Echinacea, Eyebright, Goldenseal Parsley, Barley, Lentils, Soya Beans, Split Peas, Chicken, Liver, Pork, Almonds, Brazil Nuts, cashew Nuts, Chestnuts, Hazelnuts, Macadamia Nuts, Peanuts, Pecan Nuts, Pistachio Nuts, Coconut, Walnuts, Pine Nuts, Sunflower Oil, Chocolate, Molasses, Tomato Puree, Crab, Lobster,

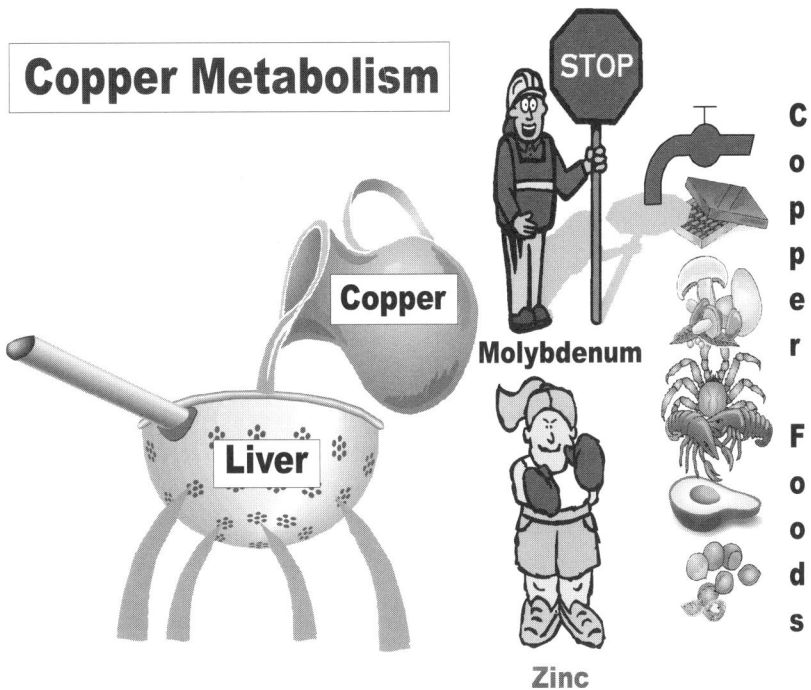

Oysters, Salmon, Kelp Sunflower Seeds Avocado, Green Beans, Beetroot, Broccoli, Fennel, Garlic, Radish, Brewer's Yeast.

But, clearly, just being on a high copper diet could not cause the results I see.

From the diagram, you can see the dynamics of copper metabolism. Copper ingestion is very easy, but there are two minerals, which limit copper absorption. These are Zinc and Molybdenum. Think of these as sentinels. What copper gets past them can always get out through the bile via the liver. However, the Xenoestrogens block the body's ability to excrete copper. Therefore Xenoestrogen exposure on a background of low zinc or low molybdenum eventually leads to copper overload because of *copper retention*.

Xenoestrogens

Pesticides (DDT, DDE, 2,4,5- T, Dieldrin,endosulfan, Arsenic, methoxychlor, kepone, toxafene, chloropicrin lindane, chlordane, artrazine)

Petroleum products (PCB's, methyl benzine, toluene, car fumes)

Plastics (PVC, lunch wraps, etc)

Hormones a. From Doctors (OCP & HRT)
b. From Food 1) Poultry industry
2) Antibiotics in animal feed

65

Zinc, Cadmium and Mercury: biology caught in the crossfire

The field of Nutritional Medicine includes toxicology. This means that there must be some awareness

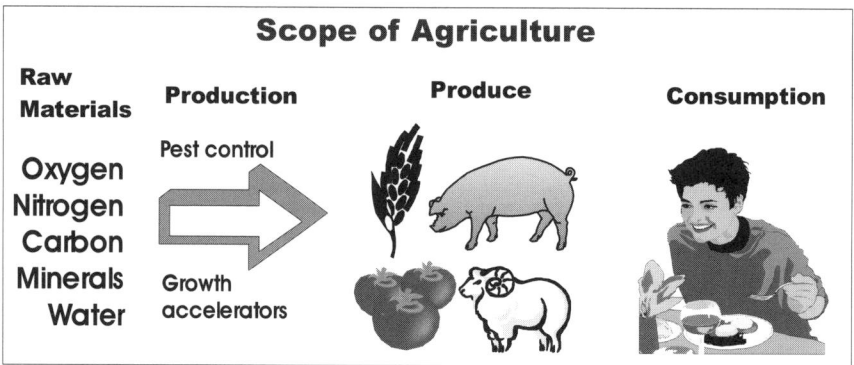

of how toxins might enter the food chain. In order to find answers, we must look at agriculture and the process of production. From raw materials, there is a series of events that transpire in order for the consumer to get edible produce. Below is a diagram depicting this.

The problem all biological systems have is that members of the "zinc series" of the periodic table are interchangeable by plants and animals. That means that if a plant is faced with zinc and cadmium

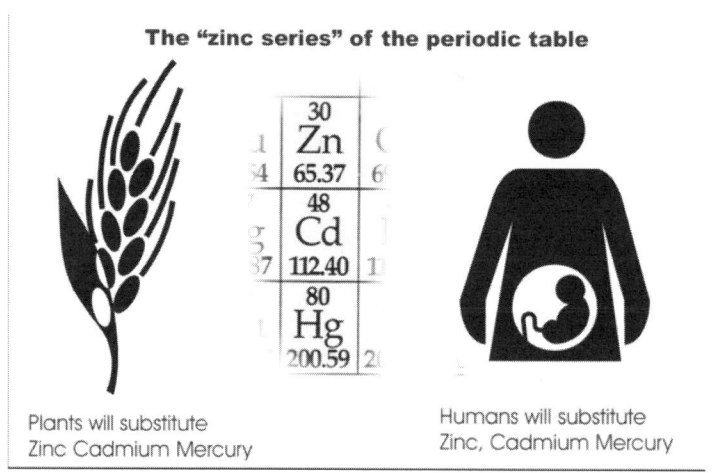

it will take up both because of the similarity of atomic structure.

Unfortunately, our superphosphate fertilisers contain about 20mg per kg of cadmium as an unavoidable contaminant. This makes cadmium present in foods fertilised this way and is a good reason for changing to organically grown food.

Other sources of cadmium are listed below in both domestic and occupational sources.

Sources of Cadmium

Domestic

Tap water
Cigarettes
Coffee, Black teas
Nuts
Refined carbohydrates
Evaporated milk
Processed meats
Organ meats
Oysters
Food grown with superphosphates fertilizers such as wheat
Industrial contamination of air and drinking water
Black rubber tyres (cars, bicycles and toys)
Pesticides
Fungicides (for tea, coffee, nuts, tobacco plants)
Paint pigments
Plastic tapes
Polyvinyl plastics (PVC's) the piping in most modern housing
Rubber carpet backing
Burned motor oil
Silver polish

Occupational

Cadmium alloys
Jewellery
Nickel-cadmium batteries
Process engraving
Soldering
Copper refining
Rust proofing tools
Marine hardware
Electroplating

This type of antagonism will occur at the tissue level with very small, amounts of either heavy metal. Toxicity as defined by industry is NOT relevant when describing focal tissue antagonism of zinc by cadmium and mercury.

This is why any examination of zinc levels must include the Antinutrients such as Cadmium and Mercury in order to fully analyse the zinc symptoms.

Sources of mercury.

Domestic sources

Body talcs and powders, Contaminated seafood, Cosmetics, Dental amalgam, Grains treated with fungicides, Fabric softeners, Fungicides used on lawns, trees & shrubs, Pesticides, Photo engraving & Wood preservatives. Vaccines (as the preservative Thiomersol). Mercurochrome

Occupational sources

Battery makers, Boiler makers, Dental nurses, Electroplates, Lamp makers, Mirror makers, Paint makers, Seed & Seedling handlers, Textile printers & Thermometer makers, canvas makers. Fluorescent Lights. Chlorine production.

The final point is this. Biology is the rope being tugged at by two forces (not always in opposition however). Until this changes, we will still see toxins in our community.

What happens to the TMA after treatment has begun? There are several points to make about this time course. Toxic elements may be under represented (smaller in TMA level than in body tissues). This is often said about Methylmercury. However, an effective detox system *will* dislodge methyl mercury and it *will* show upon subsequent TMA's. Same with hidden copper overload. One way of thinking about this is the analogy of a dam across a river. The dam might let some "overflow" of water trickle down the spillway. In times of abundance or catharsis, a lot more water may be released.

In the first TMA, toxins may be under-represented

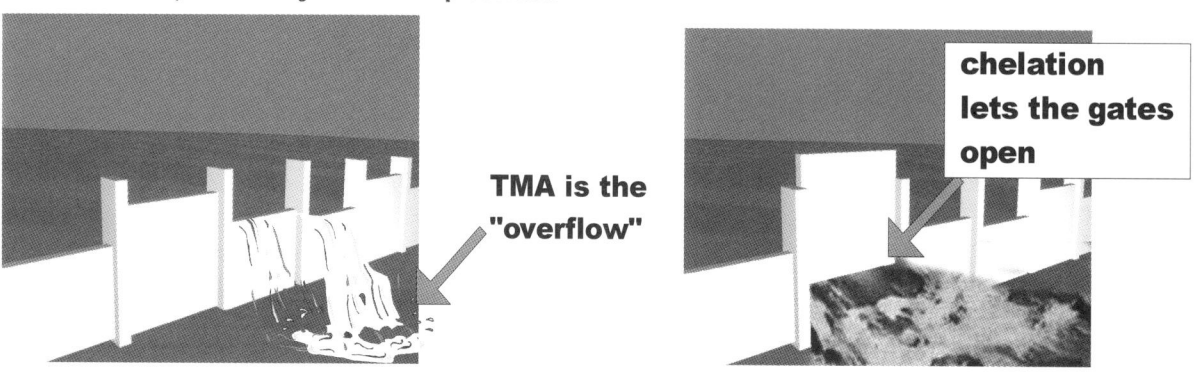

The same follows for copper and heavy metals.

Another aspect to this is that there are 2 patterns of healing. Resolution by "crisis" and resolution by

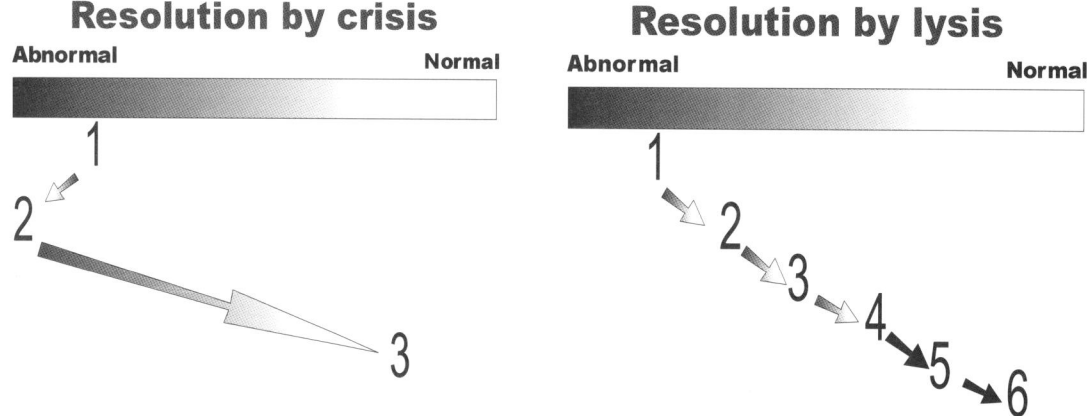

"lysis". STMA shows both of these patterns, sometimes in the one patient.
Generally speaking toxins force nutrient minerals high above the reference range. Sometime these toxins are obvious; sometimes we have to wait for the next TMA to "flush out the enemy". What we also wait for are the nutrient levels out of range to return to the reference range. In transition TMA's one may find Zinc, molybdenum or selenium drop in the TMA, even though these are being given. The analogy here is to think of these as sacrificed for the "cause" of detox.

In the case of potassium, this frequently drops very low during copper detoxification. There 2 reasons for this. The first is that potassium is important for charge integrity (balancing ions) inside cells. It carries a "one-plus" charge. Copper levels affect intracellular charge because of its "two-plus" charge. Sudden changes in copper levels may affect intracellular charge "calculations" and so the potassium drops. The second reason is that the patient always had a Channelopathy and the drop in potassium is the first sign "coming through". The take home message is that giving potassium won't really fix it.

Minerals may "fall" because they are "sacrificed"

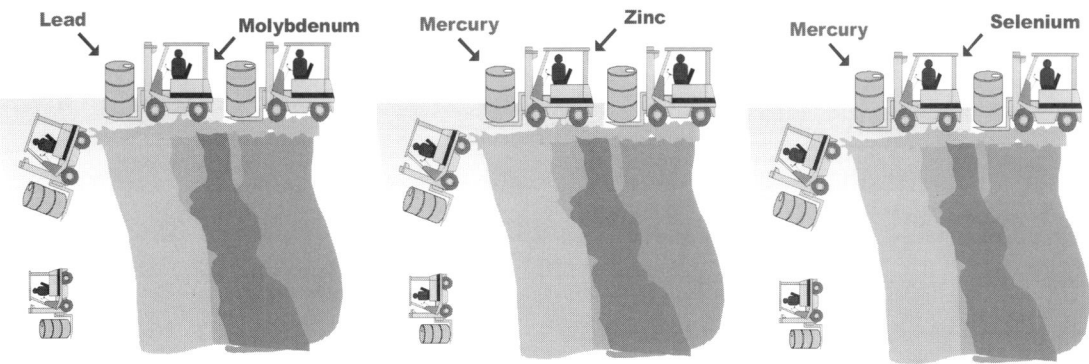

The "layers" theory. The last point to mention about STMA is that the final journey of detoxification will be a very individual path. One way to imagine this is to think of 2 processes in the sequestration of toxins. The first involved is time. Like rings of a tree, tell when there was fire or drought in a tree's life, we too go through periods of toxin exposure in our lives. The second aspect is where did the toxins go? Some tissues bind toxins more avidly, some have a higher affinity for certain metals. The levels are not homogenous in the body or even within tissue groups. Add these two effects, and final "excavation" will be unique for all (even identical twins). The sequence below (toxic elements only shown for clarity) depicts such a journey in an adult over a 2-year detox program. Persistence pays off!

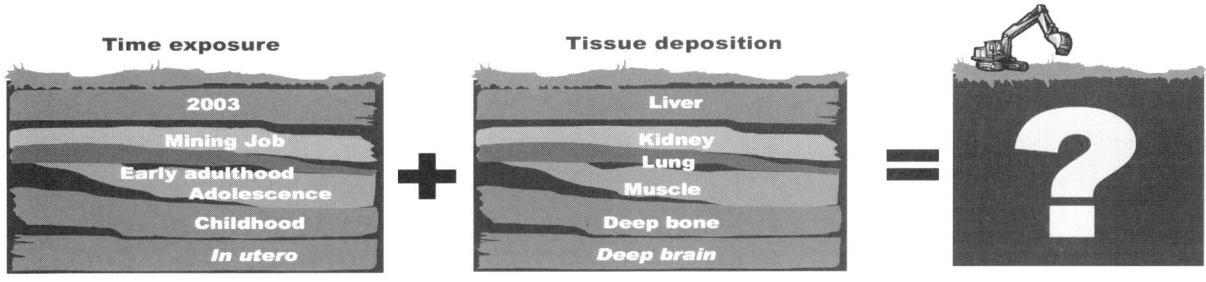

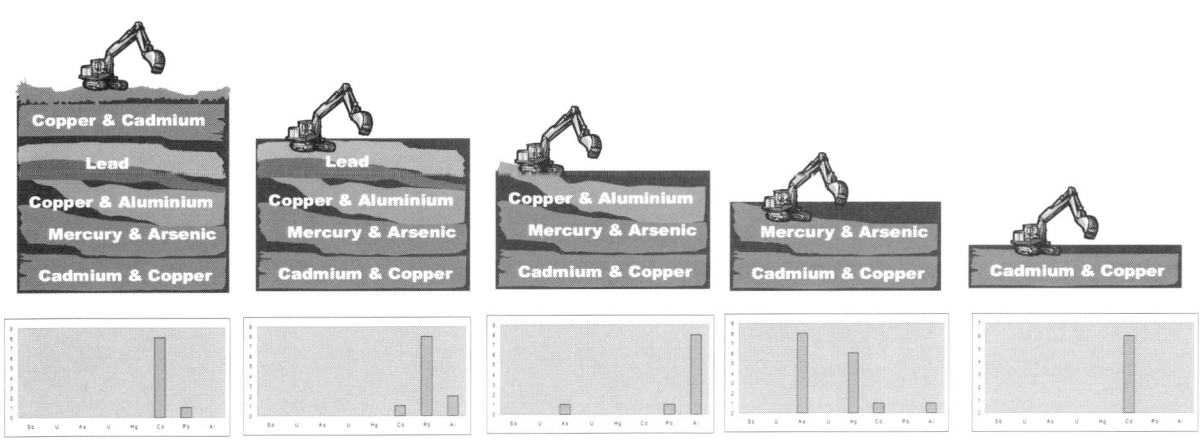

69